VITAMIN B-3 & SCHIZOPHRENIA

Other books by Dr Abram Hoffer

How To Live with Schizophrenia
(with Dr Humphry Osmond)

*Common Questions about Schizophrenia
and Their Answers*

*Hoffer's Laws of Natural Nutrition:
A Guide to Eating Well for Pure Health*

*Dr Hoffer's A,B,C of
Natural Nutrition for Children*

*Vitamin C & Cancer:
Discovery, Recover, Controversy*
(with Linus Pauling)

*Smart Nutrients:
A Guide to Nutrients that Can Prevent
and Reverse Senility*
(with Dr Morton Walker)

*Orthomolecular Nutrition:
New Lifestyle for Super Good Health*

Orthomolecular Medicine for Physicians

VITAMIN B-3 & SCHIZOPHRENIA

DISCOVERY
RECOVERY
CONTROVERSY

by Dr Abram Hoffer

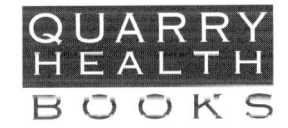

QUARRY HEALTH BOOKS

*To the thousands of my schizophrenic patients
who taught me so much and worked so hard
to recover from this disabling disease.*
— ABRAM HOFFER

Copyright © Abram Hoffer, 1998.
All rights reserved.

The publisher does not advocate the use of any particular treatment program, but believes that the information presented in this book should be available to the public. The nutritional, medical, and health information presented in this book is based on the research, training, and personal experiences of the author, and is true and complete to the best of the author's knowledge. However, this book is intended only as an informative guide for those wishing to know more about good health. It is not intended to replace or countermand the advice given by the reader's physician. Because there is always some risk involved, the author and publisher are not responsible for any adverse effects or consequences resulting from any of the suggestions made in this book. And because each person and each situation is unique, the author and the publisher urge the reader to consult with a qualified health professional before using any procedure where there is a question as to its appropriateness. It is a sign of wisdom, not cowardice, to seek a second or third opinion.

The publisher gratefully acknowledges the support of The Canada Council and the Department of Canadian Heritage for the arts of writing and publishing.

ISBN 1-55082-079-6

Design by Susan Hannah.

Printed and bound in Canada
by AGMV/Marquis, Inc., Quebec.

Published by Quarry Press Inc.,
P.O. Box 1061, Kingston, Ontario
K7L 4Y5 Canada www.quarrypress.com

CONTENTS

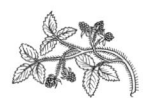

FOREWORD

The History of Treating Schizophrenia 8
Orthomolecular Psychiatry 10
Medical Ignorance 15
New Hope for Schizophrenics 17

DISCOVERY

Schizophrenia 50 Years Ago 24
The Osmond-Smythies Hypothesis 28
Vitamin B-3 35
Pilot Studies of Vitamin B-3 38
First Double-Blind Study 45
Clinical Studies 51
Project 120 53
Follow-up Studies 54
Chronic Patients 58
Results after Discharge 71
North Battleford Independent Study 73
Schizophrenia and Suicide 75

RECOVERY

Diagnosis 78
    The Hoffer Osmond Diagnostic (HOD) Test 79
    The Kryptopyrroluria (Mauve Factor) Test 83

Schizophrenic Syndromes 89
    Cerebral Allergies 89
    Vitamin Deficiencies 91
    Vitamin B-3 Dependency 92
    Mineral Deficiency 93
    Mineral Toxicity 93
    The Hallucinogens 94

Treatment 94
    Diet 95
    Vitamin Supplements 103
    Mineral Supplements 110
    Amino Acid Supplements 112
    Essential Fatty Acids 114
    Electroconvulsive Treatment (ECT) 114
    Drugs 115
    Psychiatric Treatment 121

Vitamin B-3 and Mentally Disturbed Children 122

CONTROVERSY

The Politics of Ideas 132
    American Psychiatric Association 132
    Medical Establishment 140
The New Medical Paradigm 144

Appendices 151
    HOD Test Questionnaire 152
    Kryptopyrroluria Test Procedure 162

Works Cited 164

Acknowledgements 166

FOREWORD

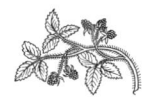

The History of Treating Schizophrenia

Orthomolecular Psychiatry

Medical Ignorance

New Hope for Schizophrenics

THE HISTORY OF TREATING SCHIZOPHRENIA

Enthusiasm for treating schizophrenia has waxed and waned over the past fifty years, and depends entirely upon the expectations of the psychiatrists. Until 1950, their expectations were nil; the previous fifty years had convinced them that nothing could be done. For this reason, they were content to warehouse patients in large institutions far from home, out of sight, but usually surrounded by beautifully-kept grounds for public display. There was a deliberate attempt to conceal from the public what was going on inside these institutions.

I still recall vividly an episode when I was about fifteen. My parents were visiting a cousin of mine who had been a long-time resident at the Saskatchewan Hospital at Weyburn. My brother, sister, and I went along with them. At the hospital we entered a very imposing front hall, with a wide, graceful staircase leading to the second floor. On the right was a private dining room for the superintendent's personal use, where he entertained friends and visiting politicians. On the left was the superintendent's large office with its private bathroom. We were all very impressed.

We were ushered into a small waiting room while the staff went to fetch our cousin. We waited and waited; I think it was at least an hour or more. Eventually our cousin arrived and we had our visit. But the long wait puzzled me, and continued to puzzle me, and continued to puzzle me until I began to visit Dr Osmond at the same hospital. He told me that the previous policy had been that no visitors were allowed to visit on the wards — they were too awful to be seen by the public. When the nurses went to bring our cousin, they first had to give him a bath and then clothes, so that we would not see him in his usual hospital garb, which was dirty and torn. After our visit he would have been returned to the ward and given back his rags — the better clothing removed, presumably, for the next visitor. The first major step forward in reforming the Saskatchewan Hospital system was to throw those wards open to the public, so they would no longer tolerate that kind of treatment of patients.

Attitudes changed about 1950. Psychiatry became more optimistic about treating schizophrenia. There was an influx of physicians into psychiatry and psychoanalysis, and dynamic psychotherapy became very influential, eventually spreading into the field. Also, insulin coma and ECT (electroconvulsive therapy) had proven that patients could get well, even if it only lasted months, rather than years.

But the main factor in the change of attitude was the introduction of tranquilizers by a French surgeon, who first showed that antihistamines were remarkable sedatives. Tranquilizers, for the first time, provided a method for calming schizophrenic patients; they cooled "hot" symptoms. Suddenly all the psychosocial theorists came into their element. It is impossible to do psychotherapy with an agitated, paranoid patient who is concentrating more on voices only he can hear than on the voice of the therapist, or to discuss problems with a patient so depressed she cannot even talk or listen. The same patient on tranquilizers or antidepressants was now "cool" and could participate in psychotherapy. Soon, armies of psychiatrists, psychologists, and social workers were happily giving psychotherapy to tranquilized patients. Drug companies wisely promoted these drugs as aids to psychotherapy, and a wave of enthusiasm swept through psychiatry.

In reality, it was a wave of over-enthusiasm which was not warranted by the facts, and it led to a mass migration of patients from institutions to alternate places, including the streets. Today, perhaps half of the homeless in North American cities are mental patients, most of them having been discharged from the hospitals. On tranquilizers, with or without psychotherapy, patients are better — their symptoms cool down — but they do not recover. A revolving door phase of therapy resulted, with patients having multiple admissions. With each admission they would be put on tranquilizers, cooled down, and then discharged. After discharge most would discontinue their medication, they would relapse, and then would have to be readmitted.

Now a counter-reaction has set in. Prominent psychiatrists who enthusiastically supported deinstitutionalization are now equally vocal in describing what a bad plan it was. Negativism is returning to psychiatry, and most psychiatrists today are content if their patients are getting by in the community on medication, and are not in hospital. They do not see recoveries, nor do they expect to see them.

Orthomolecular psychiatrists such as I do see recoveries and expect many more. Our attitude is much more optimistic, and this feeling is transmitted to patients and their families. Optimism by itself will not cure, but it will ensure patients keep on their therapeutic program, and if the family is optimistic, they will be much more patient. It is just as important to treat patients with cancer optimistically. One of the main complaints I hear from patients about cancer clinics is that they always leave feeling worse than before they went there. A recent patient complained to me that she left the clinic convinced they were preparing her for death. Schizophrenic patients do not complain about this, probably because they have never had any psychiatrist treat them with any hope or enthusiasm, but their families do.

ORTHOMOLECULAR PSYCHIATRY

By orthomolecular psychiatry I mean the use of optimum (often large) does of molecules naturally present in the body to treat poor health and to promote good health, specifically mental health. In his fundamental article on "Orthomolecular Psychiatry" published in *Science* magazine in 1968, my colleague Dr Linus Pauling stated that "orthomolecular therapy, consisting of the provision for the individual person of the optimum concentration of important normal constituents of the brain, may be the preferred treatment for many mentally ill patients." Elsewhere, he has defined orthomolecular psychiatry as "the achievement and preservation of mental health by varying concentrations in the human body of substances that are normally present, such as vitamins. It is part of a broader subject, orthomolecular medicine, an important part because the functioning of the brain is probably more sensitively dependent in its molecular composition and structure than is the functioning of other organs."

As Dr Pauling explained in his study of orthomolecular nutrition in his celebrated book *Vitamin C and the Common Cold*, the human body has lost its ability during evolution to make certain nutrients. This precept is the basis of my two books on nutrition, *Orthomolecular Nutrition* and *Hoffer's Laws of Natural Nutrition*. About 20 million years ago, man, other primates, the guinea pig, and an Indian fruit-eating bat lost the ability to make vitamin C, Dr Pauling argues. In my opinion, man is going through a process right now when we are losing the ability to make vitamin B-3 from tryptophan. People suffering from the various schizophrenias are a group who have gone far in this direction. As diets have become less natural, more high-tech, the amount of vitamin B-3 has been lowered, and those people who no longer have the machinery for converting enough tryptophan to the vitamin are becoming sick. I have been convinced for a long time that if we were to add 100 mg of vitamin B-3 in niacinamide form to our diet for every person, there would be a major decrease in the incidence of schizophrenia and many other diseases such as hyperactivity and learning and behavioral disorders in children.

Another colleague, Dr Bernard Rimland, author of *Infantile Autism*, further explains the meaning of orthomolecular and contrasts the practice of 'orthomolecular' medicine with 'toximolecular' medicine: "'Ortho' means straight or correct and 'molecular' refers to the chemistry of the body. 'Orthomolecular' thus means correcting the chemistry of the body. To contrast the philosophies of establishment medicine and orthomolecular medicine, I have coined the word 'toximolecular' to refer to the common practice of trying to treat disease (or at least the symptoms of disease) through the use of toxic chemicals. It doesn't make much sense to me; it is dangerous, expensive, and not very effective. But it is profitable. Most vitamins are quite safe, in contrast to the drugs in widespread use which can be and all too often are lethal in large amounts. Traditional medicine consists largely of giving lethal drugs in sub-lethal amounts, it seems to me. Orthomolecular psychiatry is not only much safer, it is much more sensible. Its emphasis on the use of substances normally present in the human really makes sense."

The practice of orthomolecular medicine thus recognizes that most acute and chronic diseases are due to a metabolic fault which is correctable in most patients by good nutrition, including the use of large doses of vitamins and mineral supplements. In sharp contrast, drugs are synthetics which are not naturally present in the body and for which the body does not have ready made mechanisms for their destruction and elimination. They are called xenobiotics — that is, foreign molecules. And unlike conventional medicine, orthomolecular medicine recognizes the principle of individuality in recommending the optimum diet of nutrients for each of us. No two patients are the same; no two treatments are the same. Orthomolecular medicine requires the application of both these principles, individuality and the use of optimum doses (large doses if needed) of vitamins, minerals, amino and essential fatty acids.

During the early 1950s, my colleague Dr Humphry Osmond and I developed a unified hypothesis of schizophrenia which united biochemical and psychosocial factors. We suggested that in schizophrenia there was an abnormal production of adrenochrome which then acted on the brain much as does the hallucinogen d-lysergic acid diethylamide (LSD). Adrenochrome is one of the more reactive derivatives of adrenalin. Noradrenochrome is the derivative from noradrenalin. Over the next ten years our research group in Saskatchewan established that adrenochrome is in fact an hallucinogen, that the biochemical conditions necessary for its formation in the body were all present (adrenochrome is now known to be made in the body), and that using a compound that blocked its activity on the brain was therapeutic for schizophrenia. That compound was vitamin B-3, either nicotinic acid (niacin) or nicotinamide (niacinamide).

In the orthomolecular treatment of schizophrenia, there have been two major changes over the past forty years. First, orthomolecular psychiatry has evolved from a simple use of one vitamin for treating one disease to a comprehensive holistic program which includes use of many different nutrients, in combination with standard psychiatric treatment. The only thing unorthodox about it is the emphasis given to nutrition and the use of nutrients in optimum doses. Over the past decade, nutrition has become more popular, less unorthodox, in other fields, such as cancer therapy. (However, there are still groups, like the Multiple Sclerosis Society of Canada, as insistent as ever that nutrition plays no role in disease.) Such acceptance has been slow to arrive in the realm of psychiatry, however.

Second, schizophrenia is not a single disease as we once thought: it is a syndrome with each syndrome caused by different factors. This concept was foreshadowed about 100 years ago. Psychotic patients admitted to U.S. hospitals were either suffering from pellagra, general paresis of the insane, or dementia praecox. Often they were indistinguishable from each other. After the cause of pellagra was proven to be a nutritional deficiency, pellagrins were no longer called dementia praecox (later schizophrenia). The same thing happened to scorbutic schizophrenia and to G.P.I. schizophrenia. Eventually, pellagra almost vanished, as did scurvy, and penicillin destroyed the spirochaete causing G.P.I. As each syndrome's cause was identified, it was removed from the schizophrenias, leaving psychiatry with a hard core of mysterious, untreatable, schizophrenic patients.

Over the past forty years we have identified other schizophrenic syndromes. Our work with malvaria and kryptopyrrole was elaborated by Dr C. Pfeiffer, when he gave the first clear clinical description of pyrroluria or malvaria. In time, every schizophrenic with kryptopyrrole in urine will be called pyrolluriac, not schizophrenic, and treatment will be taken over by internists who are interested in metabolic treatments. Some of the other syndromes are cerebral allergies, vitamin deficiencies and dependencies, mineral deficiencies and toxicities, and a few rarer ones caused by drugs such as the hallucinogens. Each syndrome is caused by different factors, but as the clinical disease is the same, there is a final common pathway — a pathology which affects those parts of the brain which control perception and thinking. Each syndrome will require its own particular treatment. There may be an overlap of several syndromes, for example, a combination of dairy allergy and a deficiency of vitamin B-6 and zinc.

Modern orthomolecular psychiatry is the product of the research and experiences of many clinicians, chiefly in Canada and the United States. We, from Saskatchewan, contributed toward the concept of the syndromes and introduced the concept of using optimum (large) doses of nutrients for diseases which were not considered to be vitamin deficiencies. The details of treatment will vary with different practitioners. The program I will outline in this book is the one I follow. I believe most of my colleagues will agree with these broad outlines, while they may differ on the details. Fortunately, orthomolecular psychiatry has not become fossilized as happened to psychoanalysis during Freud's lifetime. We have always encouraged diversity and open-mindedness.

MEDICAL IGNORANCE

Throughout this era, orthomolecular treatment of schizophrenia has remained controversial, when not ignored. During the early 1950s Dr Humphry Osmond and I were the first psychiatrists to use large doses of vitamins systematically for any disease, in this case vitamin B-3 for schizophrenia. Dr Irwin Stone in his book *The Healing Factor: Vitamin C against Disease* (1972) later described large doses of vitamin C as "mega" doses. The term soon became popular. It played both a positive and a negative role in furthering the use of vitamins. On the positive side, it captured people's imagination, like the buzz words "megatrends" or "megabucks." The word was never scientific, nor was it ever defined. On the negative side, it created some confusion. Many people thought there was something called a 'megavitamin'. I have had patients come to me asking to be treated with these megavitamins, when they were all ready taking large doses. "Mega" meant large dose, but did not specify how large. A few critics, ignorant of the field, defined a megadose as a dose ten times as large as those recommended daily allowances (RDAs) so beloved by government agencies and others. Some physicians were fearful of the term, which to them suggested the danger of mega toxicity. The result was a refusal by many health professionals to accept or even consider the validity of our research and the effectiveness of orthomolecular therapy for almost a whole generation. The ongoing attacks on Dr Linus Pauling following the publication of *Vitamin C and the Common Cold* were only the most celebrated examples of a concerted attempt by the medical establishment to discredit orthomolecular medicine despite the demonstrable success of our treatment of disease.

Since we first used vitamin B-3 as a main treatment component for the schizophrenias in 1952, I have supervised, as Director of Psychiatric Research, Psychiatric Services Branch,

Department of Public Health, Saskatchewan, four double-blind controlled studies and continuing clinical studies. We discovered that (1) the addition of vitamin B-3 to the treatment of schizophrenic patients doubled the natural or spontaneous recovery rate, but (2) it had no immediate effect on chronic patients, though we later discovered vitamin B-3 treatment, in combination other orthomolecular therapy, effective for chronic schizophrenics. Since then there has been massive corroboration by orthomolecular physicians, especially in the United States, Canada, and Australia; my colleagues and I have treated well over 100,000 patients since 1960. The clinical evidence of the effectiveness of orthomolecular treatment has been published in various medical journals, notably in the *Journal of Orthomolecular Medicine,* but not in the standard medical journals because they have been consistently hostile to our ideas. This treatment is considered of no value by many psychiatrists, mistakenly judged pernicious by some, and is unknown to most. "The American Psychiatric Association Task Force 7 on Megavitamins and Orthomolecular Therapy in Psychiatry" in 1973 effectively quashed interest in the use of vitamins. Further, because no drug company owns a patent on the use of vitamins, they have no vested interest in promoting their utilization; the drug companies' main efforts go into promoting and nurturing their profits from the use of a variety of tranquilizers and antidepressants. Contrary to traditional medical beliefs, orthomolecular psychiatry does not discount the use of drugs, especially antidepressants, in treatment of the schizophrenias; rather, we may use tranquilizers to cool down hot symptoms or antidepressants while introducing vitamins and minerals and other nutrients which will eventually make such drug treatment unnecessary.

NEW HOPE FOR SCHIZOPHRENICS

Orthomolecular psychiatrists have reason to be hopeful in their treatment of schizophrenia. First, the treatment does work, despite the harping of medical bodies and pharmaceutical companies. And second, an increasing number of health professionals and families are turning to orthomolecular medicine when faced by the failings of conventional pharmaceutical and psychotherapeutic treatments.

This sense of hope shines through the case history of two schizophrenic patients I treated in the 1980s, Faye and John, who suffered alone for many years, met each other, married, and now get on very well together. They each received the holistic, orthomolecular therapy I advocate in this book: every treatment component was important, but only after vitamin therapy did their lives start to come together again.

Faye came to see me in June 1984, complaining she was run down and nervous. She was fifty years old. She had not been well from birth, but she told me she first broke down when she was six years old. Her mother told me there had been no breakdown at that time, but Faye could not get along with her teacher and was taken out of school. Two years earlier she had fallen on her face, smashing her nose. This was repaired, but she required more surgery when she was fifteen, and she remained sensitive about her appearance.

In 1962, she became very nervous after the birth of her son. She thought she was given a series of ECT. Following treatment, her parents took her back to Alberta to convalesce, but she did not recover and was admitted to an Alberta mental hospital for six weeks. In the years following that she had five more admissions, the last one for two months in 1981. In the meantime, her daughter was placed in a foster home because Faye was unable to care for her. Her general practitioner, in referring her to me, wrote that she was having evil thoughts; she was afraid she might hurt someone inadvertently, perhaps her mother.

A mental status examination revealed she had heard voices in the past, still heard herself think, and had hallucinated happy faces. She was more concerned about her appearance and about people, whom she believed were very critical of her. Her memory was poor and her concentration faulty. She was bothered by depression, but she was not considering suicide. She weighed 161 pounds, having come down from 220 by watching her diet. She drank three glasses of milk daily, suffered many colds and sinus discharge, and coughed a lot.

I advised her to eliminate sugar and dairy products from her diet, and added niacin (vitamin B-3) 1 gram three times per day, ascorbic acid (vitamin C) 500 mg three times a day, vitamin B-6 100 mg per day, and zinc sulfate 220 mg a day to the drugs she was already taking. Her medications included chlorpromazine 200 mg daily, imap 2 mg i.m. every week, and parnate 20 mg a day.

I saw her again in September 1984, by which time she had shown some improvement. Her skin was healthier, her sinuses were clear, her weight was now 150, her fears were gone, she was no longer paranoid, and her memory was better. Parnate was making her nauseated so I asked her to discontinue it.

In mid-November she was given a vaccination against flu and soon after began to suffer headaches. She became paranoid again, but had no hallucinations. She was admitted to hospital from December 24, 1984, to January 5, 1985. She remained on niacin and ascorbic acid, plus chlorpromazine 250 mg daily and imap. For the next three months she was very disturbed. I stopped her imap and replaced it with another tranquilizer, fluanxol 40 mg i.m. every seven days.

In July 1985 she complained how lonely she was, even in a group home. Her son and daughter visited her regularly. She was now convinced milk made her sick because whenever she had some she became nauseated. I started her on anafranil 50 mg before bed, but it made her worse and was therefore discontinued. By August 1985 she was at last completely dairy-free. She was now receiving 500 mg per day of chlorpromazine.

On November 25, 1985, she told me she had missed two injections. She was confused and very paranoid. I admitted her to hospital until December 7, 1985. The fluanxol was stopped and she was started on modecate 25 mg i.m. weekly.

On May 14, 1986, her situation was much better. She was free of hallucinations, was not paranoid, and her mood was good. She was down to 150 mg of chlorpromazine a day. However, by August 1986 she was worse again, and had begun to see faces in the rug. October 30, 1986, I stopped her modecate and started haldol injections, 300 mg once a month. She switched her vitamin B-3 from niacin to niacinamide.

In July 1987 she remained nervous and restless, but she was much better. She had started to read about schizophrenia because she was worried about her son. She was also doing volunteer work, which she enjoyed. For the rest of 1987 and 1988 she fluctuated, now and then being depressed or nervous, and sometimes having more hallucinations.

In January 1989 she was cheerful, and two months later, in March, married Jim, a schizophrenic, unemployed, age forty eight. They had met at the group home where they both lived. After they married, they began to look for an apartment of their own. Faye's chlorpromazine was now 250 mg per day. By August 1989 she still hallucinated occasionally.

At the end of 1989 I discontinued her parenteral haldol and gave her 10 mg per day of the oral haldol tablets. She learned to adjust the dose to control her nervousness, and by the end of 1990 was feeling stable. This patient had called my office at least three times a week for several years, but in December 1990 there were no calls until around Christmas, when she called to report she was getting on well.

Faye and Jim's marriage worked out well. They support each other, and because they understand the illness, they are very tolerant of each other's symptoms. They remind each other about their medication and vitamins. I consider Faye much improved. That is, she is getting on well in the community, gets on well with her family, and is mostly free of symptoms. She is unable to work because her life had been disrupted too much, for too long, and she will require medical help for the rest of her life, but she is content, often cheerful, and has established a new life with a man with whom she is compatible.

Jim first came to see me in June 1989, after he and Faye were married. Since then I have seen them together about every two or three months. Jim had become sick during his teens. He had been in hospital at age fourteen for eight months, again in 1973, and for the last time in 1977, when he was thirty-six years old. Since then he had taken his drugs carefully. He was on parenteral modecate 25 mg every ten days, xanax, chlorpromazine, and medication for high blood pressure. I added niacin and ascorbic acid, 3 grams of each per day, to his program. In December 1989 I decreased the niacin to 500 mg three times a day and added the same amount of niacinamide. In November 1990, he told me he felt like a "million bucks." He remained on his parenteral tranquilizer and vitamins. Their marriage was working out well.

No one expected them ever to marry, much less to enter into a happy, successful marriage. Schizophrenic patients, when sick, find it impossible to have successful relationships. The fact that Faye and Jim's marriage is working out so well is another measure of how much they have improved.

Despite their remarkable improvement in health, Faye and Jim will be permanent charges to society, and rightly so, for they are victims of a psychiatric care system which seems incapable of accepting truly new ideas. Faye had been ill twenty-two years before I saw her; Jim had been ill since age fourteen. It is highly improbable either one was going to improve spontaneously. Both would be expected to remain dependent and ill, with the occasional re-admission to hospital to adjust their medication. Ideally, Jim and Faye should not have had to wait so long before they were started on effective treatment, for Faye could have been started on vitamin B-3 when she first became ill. Jim, too, could have been started on treatment when he was fourteen. At the beginning of their illnesses they would have responded much more quickly; they would have been spared an enormous amount of ill health, pain and suffering, and disruption of their lives. Society would have been spared the cost of looking after them for the rest of their lives.

Still, there is hope these ideas can be properly disseminated, which is the reason I have written *Vitamin B-3 & Schizophrenia: Discovery, Recovery, Controversy*. This belief was reinforced for me by a patient I saw in December 1990. He was a young man who was first treated for schizophrenia at University Hospital, Saskatoon, with several admissions, the last in June 1990. One brother was schizophrenic in a mental hospital in Vancouver, British Columbia. His mother read the small book Dr Osmond and I wrote in 1966, based on our research with vitamin B-3 treatments, *How To Live with Schizophrenia*, on the advice of her brother-in-law, Dan. I had treated Dan for schizophrenia over thirty years ago in Saskatoon. After three years of treatment Dan became well; he has remained well to this day. He became a school teacher, and is now successfully operating several business ventures. He fulfils one of my main criteria for recovery; that is, the ability to pay taxes. Dan spoke to his nephew about schizophrenia and encouraged him to see me. There will not be many other Dans until information about orthomolecular treatment of schizophrenia is more widely read and orthomolecular psychiatry is more widely practiced.

DISCOVERY

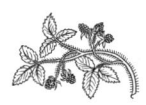

Schizophrenia 50 Years Ago

The Osmond-Smythies Hypothesis
(The Mauve Factor)

Vitamin B-3

Pilot Studies

First Double-Blind Study

Clinical Studies

Project 120

Follow-Up Studies

Chronic Patients

Results after Discharge

North Battleford Independent Study

Schizophrenia and Suicide

SCHIZOPHRENIA 50 YEARS AGO

In 1950, schizophrenia had been described clinically and categorized so well that modern descriptions have really not improved much over what we knew then. There was no specific treatment, and what treatment we had yielded results not much better than those achieved in England by J. Conolly in 1850, as reported in his *An Inquiry Concerning the Indications of Insanity*. The treatments included restraint; i.e., forced stay in hospital, sometimes restraint within the hospital such as locked rooms, most often locked wards, and occasionally restraint garments. It also included electroconvulsive therapy (ECT) and sedative drugs. ECT was helpful to many patients for brief periods, but in most cases it was followed by relapse. Insulin coma was rapidly falling into disfavor because it was dangerous and did not yield permanent recoveries. It was said that of all early patients, one-third recovered spontaneously, one-third became repeaters, and one-third remained ill. Psychotherapy was very popular and was given to schizophrenics when staff was available. The results were dismal. Patients who failed to respond within a period of months were sent to a mental hospital where they often stayed for years, if not forever. These hospitals were already too full of chronic patients, who had been accumulating for many years.

Patients and families were given no information about the illness, which remained mysterious. Psychiatry's paranoid tendency of blaming parents and society for the illness was just beginning to take hold. Families were devastated by the illness. The first major attempt to describe the disease with a spirit of hope did not appear until 1966 with our book, *How To Live with Schizophrenia*. Without doubt, schizophrenia was the single most devastating disease. About half of all hospital beds were occupied by schizophrenic patients. Even today, each young schizophrenic will cost his or her community between $1-2 million over a lifetime of illness, because even with tranquilizers the patient will not recover. Schizophrenia was our major challenge as psychiatrists in the 1950s.

In 1951, the number of centers worldwide doing research in psychiatry could be counted on one's fingers — perhaps we would need a few toes — but Saskatchewan was not one of them. At the Allan Memorial Hospital, under Professor Ewan Cameron, McGill University had the most active research program, followed probably by the University of Toronto Medical College. A little was done in Halifax at Dalhousie University, but I cannot recall any studies originating from elsewhere in Canada. Verdun Protestant Hospital in Montreal, now Douglas Hospital, was beginning some clinical research, but the drugs it helped introduce were known in France only.

This poor distribution of effort bothered Dr C. Roberts, head of psychiatry for the Government of Canada in Ottawa, who was in charge of research grants. The Government of Canada had assigned money to be used for psychiatric research, so much per person. Ontario and Quebec were using the money they were entitled to, but none of the four western provinces were. This may have been the main reason why we in Saskatchewan were given our first grant of $23,000 in 1952.

In 1950 I had completed my internship at City Hospital, Saskatoon. I had gone into medicine after receiving my PhD in agricultural biochemistry from the University of Minnesota in 1944. During my internship I became very interested in psychiatry, especially psychosomatic medicine: so many patients had vague, long-standing complaints which did not conform to the acute syndromes we had studied in medical school. Hoping to combine research, medicine, and psychiatry, I approached Dr D. C. McKerracker, Chief, Psychiatric Services Branch, Department of Public Health. He was the second major factor in creating the research unit in Saskatchewan.

In 1950 I joined the Department of Public Health as a resident in psychiatry at the Munro Wing of Regina General Hospital, and was also given grant support to help establish research. But my most important work was to learn psychiatry. There was no medical school: we learned from our patients, from senior psychiatrists, from the nurses (who knew more than we did), and from our reading. At regular intervals, well-known psychiatrists such as Dr Karl Menninger would be invited to give us days or weeks of seminars. Primarily, however, we learned by doing. After I had gained my certificate as specialist in psychiatry, I would have more time to start a research program. Dr McKerracker agreed with this, and he was given support by psychiatrists in eastern Canada with whom he had discussed this. Professor A. Stokes, University of Toronto, agreed it would be a good idea for Saskatchewan to start a research program.

Dr McKerracker had been brought to Saskatchewan by a new government. The Premier, Mr. T. C. "Tommy" Douglas, had once worked for a few months as a minister intern at Saskatchewan Hospital in Weyburn, and he had been appalled by what he had seen. Premier Douglas later became the champion of the now famous "medicare" system of public health care and insurance in Saskatchewan and then Canada as the leader of the New Democratic Party. But at the time Saskatchewan had one of the worst mental health care systems in the western world. Even in 1954, Dr John Weir, Medical Director, Rockefeller Foundation, classed our hospitals as among the three worst he had ever seen. The other two were in Egypt and Jamaica. Dr McKerracker was given the job of bringing Saskatchewan psychiatry into the twentieth century.

The third psychiatrist who made our research possible was Dr Humphry Osmond. He had been recruited by Dr McKerracker to become Superintendent of the Saskatchewan Hospital, Weyburn. Dr Osmond had become unhappy with the state of British psychiatry and its lack of opportunity for him to carry on research. He had applied to Saskatchewan thinking he would have freedom of action. With Dr John Smythies, Dr Osmond had hypothesized that there was a toxic compound, an "M" substance, in schizophrenics, which was somehow analogous to adrenalin, with the properties of mescaline, the hallucinogen. They had compared the psychological experience induced by mescaline in normal people and the schizophrenic experience, and had also realized that mescaline was a phenylethyl amine, similar in structure to adrenalin. They had also observed that, in a few subjects, deteriorated (discolored) adrenalin solutions as used by asthmatics often caused the same kind of experience.

I met Dr Osmond in the fall of 1951, the same day he arrived in Regina after a long train trip across Canada. He had with him the manuscript he and Dr Smythies had written. This began our long, friendly, collegial relationship, and we began to forge the research program for which Saskatchewan became well-known. It required the combined interests of three of us: Dr McKerracker, Dr Osmond, and me. There were several other essential preconditions: the massive interest of the Government of Saskatchewan to improve their health care system, and the absence of a medical school in Saskatchewan. Had there been a medical college, it would have had a department of psychiatry staffed by psychiatrists eager to become psychoanalysts, who would have rejected any biochemical approach toward the study of schizophrenia. I am not being unfair; in 1950, in Canada and the United States, the departments of psychiatry of every medical college were staffed by this type of psychiatrist. By 1954, most young psychiatrists hoped to become analysts, and regretted it if they could not. In 1954 in the United States, it was almost impossible to become a professor of psychiatry without having undergone personal psychoanalysis. In North America, medical colleges have not been noted for the quality of their psychiatric research programs. In brief, we started in Saskatchewan because there were three of us who were interested, and because there was minimal opposition to our ideas.

THE OSMOND-SMYTHIES HYPOTHESIS
(The Mauve Factor)

With the introductory work of Osmond and Smythies, it became possible to tackle this dreadful disease. Osmond and Smythies' toxin "M" hypothesis provided us with a set of directions for searching the body for a schizophrenic toxin. To isolate any substance, one must have a property or trait which is associated with the compound. For example, it was found that rice bran or whole rice would cure beriberi in pigeons. One could then fractionate the rice and test each fraction for its anti-beriberi properties. Fractions, which were more potent, would contain more of the compound, now known to be thiamine. In this way, pure crystalline thiamine was isolated and its structure then determined. But to isolate a schizophrenic toxin was impossible if its only property was to cause schizophrenia. It could not really be tested in animals, nor given to human subjects. However, compounds which reproduced some of the features of schizophrenia could be tested. Another way would be to examine every known compound in the body, but this would not help either, as no scientist would even start such an enormous task.

As soon as I read Osmond and Smythies' manuscript I realized that, if properly exploited, this idea could lead us to the toxin "M." At the same time, I urged Humphry to publish his paper as soon as possible so that his priority on the idea would be established. He submitted it to the *British Mental Journal*, whose editor, Dr Fleming, promptly accepted it for publication, even though Dr Smythies had become ambivalent about seeing it in print.

The Osmond-Smythies hypothesis was based on the

fact that each chemical molecule is unique. However, molecules which are similar in structure share some properties while displaying differences. Thus, all tricyclic antidepressants have similar antidepressant properties while differing in dosages required and side effects or toxicity. The Osmond-Smythies hypothesis suggested we search the body for a substance with the psychological properties of mescaline and similar in structure to adrenalin, a catecholamine, as are noradrenalin and dopamine. This idea arose from their observation that pink (deteriorated) adrenalin was, in some people, an hallucinogen. The word "hallucinogen" was then not in use. It was first used by Dr Don Johnson, a British M.P., in one of his monographs on the hallucinogens.

I began to collect information on all the compounds then known to be hallucinogenic, which we defined as compounds that produced a mescaline-type reaction without changes in levels of consciousness, which excluded anaesthetics, for example. The list was short. It included d-lysergic acid diethylamide (d-LSD-25), harmline, mescaline, ibogaine, and deteriorated adrenalin. To my amazement and excitement, they were all indoles (LSD, harmline, ibogaine), or could become indoles (mescaline). We did not know what pink adrenalin was.

Our new guidelines or directions in looking for the schizophrenic toxin were now more specific: look for an indole which was related to adrenalin and was an hallucinogen. This simple guideline decreased the number of potential toxins from hundreds to a mere handful. However, we did not know what this new indole was until Professor D.E. Hutcheon told us at the first meeting of the Saskatchewan Committee on Schizophrenia Research in 1952. He had gotten his PhD under Professor Burns at Oxford with his dissertation on adrenochrome — a red compound formed by the oxidation of adrenalin. It fuses the side chain to the six carbon ring to form an indole. Our potential schizophrenic toxin was adrenochrome, an indole derived by the oxidation of adrenalin. All the catecholamines are oxidized readily to their respective indoles, thus noradrenalin to noradrenochrome, dopamine to dopachrome. In 1952 hardly anything was known about these reactions. It was known that adrenal glands, when cut open, would turn red on standing in air, and that adrenalin unprotected by antioxidants would turn pink, then red, later brown, and finally black. My first professor of biochemistry, Roger Manning, in 1936 published one of the few papers on adrenochrome, but in 1951 I was unaware of this.

Our final equations were:

1. noradrenalin ———> adrenalin
2. adrenalin ———> adrenochrome

We knew Equation 1 required methyl groups, which are provided by methyl donors. Noradrenalin is a methyl acceptor. It picks up one methyl group to become adrenalin. We knew nothing about Equation 2.

To establish some validity to this hypothesis that adrenochrome was involved in the etiology of schizophrenia, we had to find out the following:

∾ 1. What influenced Reaction 1? How could it be increased or inhibited? For increasing the amount of adrenalin could increase the production of adrenochrome, which would either cause or be harmful to schizophrenics, while decreasing the reaction would be therapeutic.

∾ 2. Factors affecting Reaction 2 are more relevant. We knew little about this except that it occurred spontaneously in pure solution and in air. It was an oxidation reaction which would be accelerated by oxidants and inhibited or prevented by antioxidants, more commonly known as reducing substances. Nothing was known about the formation of adrenochrome in the body.

⁂ 3. It was very important to determine the properties of adrenochrome, whether in fact adrenochrome was an hallucinogen. It would be essential to find out what it did in the body, which enzymes were affected, and how to reverse the reaction.

⁂ 4. These were all important questions, but we knew even if these reactions were true, it would take years and decades to establish. In the meantime, we desperately needed better treatment for schizophrenia. We decided to assume the reactions were correct and to develop chemical treatments which were a logical offshoot from our adrenochrome hypothesis; i.e., to use chemicals which would decrease the formation of adrenochrome and/or would act as an antidote.

There were two ways of shutting down the formation of adrenochrome. We could divert the adrenalin to other compounds rather than allowing it to go to adrenochrome. If we could prevent the addition of methyl groups to noradrenalin, then less adrenalin would be available for forming adrenochrome. To do so we decided to try vitamin B-3. I knew something about vitamins, having studied them while doing the research on vitamins in cereal products during my PhD education at the University of Minnesota. Four natural methyl acceptors are now known — thiamin (vitamin B-1), riboflavin (vitamin B-2), niacin (vitamin B-3), and ubiquinone (coenzyme Q 10). Then, however, few methyl acceptors were known. Coenzyme Q 10 was not known then and the vitamins B-1 and B-2 were not as clearly related to psychosis as vitamin B-3 was. Vitamin B-3 was readily available and it was the safest and easiest to administer.

Both forms of vitamin B-3, niacin and niacinamide, are

methyl acceptors — that is, they pick up methyl groups. We thought that this vitamin might decrease the formation of adrenalin by making less nor adrenalin available. The process of adding and removing methyl groups from molecules is called transmethylation. In 1952 transmethylation had not been established as a normal reaction in the body. We also knew that vitamin B-3 was the anti pellagra vitamin, that it had been used in large doses for treating some organic confusional conditions and some patients with depression, and that it was safe to use even in large doses. In the body, vitamin B-3 is converted into nicotinamide adenine dinucleotide, which is present in both oxidized (NAD) and reduced forms (NADH). But this coenzyme is involved in many reactions in the body involving oxidation reduction in the respiratory chain. It is involved in over 200 reactions in the body.

Vitamin B-3 was then one of the few methyl receptors known. In fact, after the last world war liver damage caused by methyl deficiency was a favorite medical problem. This even made it difficult to use vitamin B-3 because immediately questions arose about damage to the liver. Early studies giving large amounts of vitamin B-3 to animals suggested there were serious changes in liver — it became filled with fat. However, research we did several years later proved these early results were wrong. In our research, giving the same amount of vitamin B-3 to the same animals species showed no pathological changes to be present. Vitamin B-3, therefore, by diverting methyl groups could decrease the formation of adrenalin. Whether it does do so remains unknown.

Vitamin B-3 does decrease the formation of adrenochrome in the brain. The oxidation of adrenalin to adrenochrome takes place in two steps. In the first step, the adrenalin loses one electron to form what has been called oxidized adrenalin. It is a very reactive molecule. In the presence of NAD and NADH, it recaptures one electron once more to form adrenalin and this reaction keeps on going back and forth. But if there is not sufficient NAD and NADH, the oxidized adrenalin loses another electron to become adrenochrome. This can no longer be changed back to adrenalin. Thus, in the absence of vitamin B-3, one of the precursors of NAD, more adrenochrome is formed. The same reactions occur with the other catechol amines. Noradrenalin will be changed to noradrenochrome and dopamine to dopachrome. But at the same time by decreasing the further oxidation of adrenalin to adrenochrome, it also increases the amount of adrenalin which can be used for other physiological purposes.

For example, it is now believed that Parkinsonism is caused by a deficiency of l-dopa. This is why this compound is given to these patients. What has not been taken into account is what happens to the dopamine once it has been given. I have no doubt it is converted to dopachrome and thus it has two activities. It increases the amount of l-dopa in the brain, which helps relieve these patients of some of the symptoms of their disease, but by increasing the amount of dopachrome, it will make many of them psychotic depending on the amount which is given and may, according to some medical authorities, hasten their death. Thus this drug, which is so helpful at the time, decreases life span. However, a recent report supports the finding that vitamin B-3 and coenzyme Q 10 spare dopamine. J. B. Shulz and colleagues found that in animals made to have Parkinsonism by the administration of MPTP, giving them these two natural substances protected the animals by protecting them against the dopamine depletion the toxic drug produces. Q 10 and vitamin B-3 make up what is called complex A in the respiratory chain of respiratory enzymes. I have given two Parkinsonism patients these two vitamins and it has been very effective in helping them.

Before starting any therapeutic trials, Dr Osmond and I laid down some very important specifications:

∾ 1. The chemical must be safe even when used in large amounts.

∾ 2. The optimum amount would have to be used.

∾ 3. It would have to be taken orally for a long time, perhaps forever, for we considered schizophrenia a disease more comparable to diabetes mellitus than to acute appendicitis or pneumonia. A chronic biochemical disease could respond only temporarily to treatments such as ECT whose effect was transient.

With these conditions in mind, we soon concluded that only water soluble vitamins could meet our requirements. We thus settled on vitamin B-3 and vitamin C (ascorbic acid) as the main ones we should examine.

In 1952 we were not aware of any clinical studies where more than 1.5 grams of vitamin B-3 had been used. We had not seen Dr W. Kaufman's work with arthritics reported in his *Common Form of Niacinamide Deficiency Syndrome Disease: Aniacinamidosis* (1943) and *The Common Form of Joint Dysfunction: Its Incidence and Treatment* (1949). He administered up to 4 grams daily. We concluded that had smaller doses been effective in treating schizophrenia, the pellagrologists working in mental hospitals in the mid-1930s would have observed this. It is possible they did observe something. They were impressed with the one-disease/one-deficiency school of thought; i.e., pellagra is caused by a deficiency of vitamin B-3 and, conversely, if pellagra is not present, no extra vitamin B-3 is required. They would diagnose any patient getting well on B-3 as pellagra, while patients who did not recover would remain labeled schizophrenia. We decided to use at least 3 grams per day and to go much higher if necessary. As far as we knew, vitamin C was safe, rarely caused any side effects and could be given in much larger doses. I had taken 1 gram doses as a crystalline powder several years before and had used it to counteract insect bites, even colds, but had not done any systematic studies with it.

VITAMIN B-3

(Niacin and Niacinamide)

Vitamin B-3 was the third water soluble vitamin discovered: vitamin B-1 (thiamine) was the first, and vitamin B-2 (riboflavin) was the second. In the mid-1930s researchers recognized that nicotinic acid was a vitamin. This simple chemical had been known for more than fifty years, but no one had suspected its role in nutrition. There are two chemicals with vitamin B-3 properties, nicotinic acid and nicotinamide, also referred to as niacin and niacinamide, respectively. Both are converted into co-enzyme one or nicotinamide dinucleotide (NAD).

The term "B-3" was initially used for both the niacin and the niacinamide forms of the vitamin, but not long thereafter was replaced by the proper chemical names: nicotinic acid and nicotinamide. For medical reasons these were shortened to niacin and niacinamide. Nicotinic acid reminds people of nicotine, from which it can be made. The term vitamin B-3 was again popularized by Mr. Bill Wilson (Bill W., co-founder of Alcoholics Anonymous) in a series of bulletins entitled "The Vitamin B-3 Therapy," which were widely distributed through Alcoholics Anonymous. The public found vitamin B-3 more acceptable.

Vitamin B-3 helps to control blood fat levels. It is important for the treatment of mental illness because of its effects on complex chemical interactions that affect the working of the nervous system. Vitamin B-3 is made in the body from the amino acid tryptophan. On the average 1 mg of vitamin B-3 is made from 60 mg of tryptophan, a 1.5 percent conversion rate. Since it is made in the body, it does not meet the strict definition of a vitamin, which are defined as substances that cannot be made in the body. It should have been classified with the amino acids but long association has given it permanent status a a vitamin. I suspect that one day in the far distant future none of the tryptophan in the body will be converted into vitamin B-3 and it then will truly be a vitamin.

The 1.5 percent conversion rate is a compromise based on the conversion of tryptophan to N-methyl nicotinamide and its metabolites in human subjects. The amount converted is not inflexible but varies with conditions and from patient to patient. For example, women pregnant in their last three months convert tryptophan to niacin metabolites three times as efficiently as non-pregnant females. It was observed a long time ago that pregnant women were to a degree less prone to develop schizophrenia, and when it did occur, it took the form of a post partum psychosis. In schizophrenics we suspected that there is a decrease in the production of niacin from tryptophan, the sign of a slow evolutionary change which will one day totally remove this source of niacin, and we will have to depend entirely on external sources.

The best known vitamin B-3 deficiency disease is pellagra. More accurately it is a tryptophan deficiency disease since tryptophan alone can cure the early stages. The word "cure" is actually inappropriate, because no one is ever "cured" of pellagra: as soon as our daily intake of vitamin B-3 falls to a very low level, this dreadful disease is waiting to do us in. Pellagra was endemic in the Southern United States until the beginning of the last world war. It can be described by the four D's — dermatitis, diarrhea, dementia, and death. The dementia is a late stage phenomenon. In the early stages it resembles much more the schizophrenias and can only with difficulty be distinguished from it. I consider it one of the schizophrenic syndromes.

Niacin and niacinamide are available as tablets or capsules, in dosages ranging from 50 to 500 mg per tablet. The larger dose tablets are used when gram or larger dosages are needed. The 50 and 100 mg tablets usually contain too much filler and would make most people ill if the usual 3000 mg per day were used. Niacinamide is the form usually present in multivitamin or B-complex preparations in amounts up to 100 mg. Niacin may be present, but in much lower quantities as it can cause flushing of the skin even in low doses. Small amounts of niacinamide are added to most of the white flour milled in the United States and Canada, a practice which has been effective in almost eliminating classical pellagra.

The optimum dose of vitamin B-3 varies enormously with the disease being treated, and may have to be determined by clinical trial. An average dose is started, which is in time increased or decreased depending upon the therapeutic response and side effects. The dose range for niacinamide is more restricted, and it is seldom possible to go higher than 6 grams per day because it will induce nausea and vomiting. The best dose is below this level. It is possible to go much higher with niacin, and a few patients have taken up to 60 grams per day. The optimum dose is an effective dose below the nauseant dose.

Both forms of vitamin B-3 are anti-pellagra, but only niacin will normalize cholesterol levels, lowering total and low density lipoprotein cholesterol, and elevating high density lipoprotein cholesterol, thus restoring the ratio of total to HDL cholesterol to its normal value of less than 5. At a recent meeting in Victoria, B.C., on hypercholesterolemia (high cholesterol), American internists where strongly supporting niacin and claimed they had little problem with it. They had to have an economical product or their patients could not afford it. Niacin was the treatment of choice for the poor. Canadian physicians downplayed it, for in Canada drug plans picked up all or most of the cost so they preferred the new, expensive "statins."

Only niacin causes a transient vasodilation or flush,

usually beginning in the face and working its way down the body, rarely as far as the legs and feet. The flush generally disappears altogether within a few weeks, as long as one continues to take it regularly. However, about one percent of all patients on niacinamide will also develop a flush, which is usually milder than the niacin reaction. These patients appear to convert niacinamide to niacin in their bodies quickly enough to build niacin up to a flush level.

PILOT STUDIES

Before 1950, vitamin B-3 had been given to small numbers of patients in doses up to 1.5 grams per day. These must have been considered large doses, for as an anti-pellagra compound only a few milligrams per day would be needed, and usually less than 50 mg per day would cure pellagra. Chronic pellagrins needed up to 600 mg per day, but this was not common knowledge. The few authors who tried vitamin B-3 on patients with depression found it was helpful. We knew that a proportion of patients with depression eventually turned out to be schizophrenic, so we assumed that the responders in these early studies were in the beginning stages of schizophrenia, when it is difficult to distinguish schizophrenia from simple mood disorders. We had no reason to think the vitamin could be of value to non-schizophrenic patients. Today, more than thirty-five years later, I would not reason this way, having seen many patients with depression who have responded. Recently, I saw a man on follow-up after one month on niacin who had not responded to two years of treatment, but three hours after taking 500 mg of niacin, his depression began to lift. By the time I saw him for the second time, after one month on niacin, he was nearly free of depression.

However, in 1951 we needed all the encouragement we could muster because we knew the odds against us finding a treatment for schizophrenia were 1000 to one. In 1951, any psychiatrist who thought schizophrenia might have a biochemical basis was considered an anomaly, a freak. At the first American Psychiatric Association meeting I attended in 1952, in Los Angeles, there were around 900 members. I believe I was the only one with a background or even an interest in biochemistry.

At our first meeting of the Saskatchewan Committee on Schizophrenia Research, we had agreed to start studies with the vitamins. I immediately discovered this would be difficult. For starters, only 100 mg tablets were available commercially, and we realized patients would refuse to swallow 30 pills a day in order to achieve the daily 3 gram dosage. These tablets also contained a lot of filler in order to make them large enough to swallow easily. This amount of filler (junk) could make our patients sick. This, in fact, happened fifteen years later at a large mental hospital near Los Angeles. After I made a series of presentations at this hospital, they decided to try niacin. I had recommended 500 mg tablets, but their pharmacy would provide only 100 mg tablets, which did make the patients ill, and the project never got underway.

I wrote to the pharmaceutical firm Merck and Co. (now Merck Sharp & Dohme) in Rahway, New Jersey. Merck had been manufacturing the B vitamins, issuing a series of monographs on each of their vitamins which had been very helpful to us. I told them what I hoped to do, and requested supplies of niacin, niacinamide, riboflavin, thiamine, and ascorbic acid. Within a few weeks we received 50 pound drums of each vitamin, which were turned over to the hospital dispensary. The dispensary agreed to make up 500 mg capsules, and these were placed in bottles of 200, one month's supply. Our first studies were done using these pure vitamins. Later, when we planned our double blind controlled experiment, we requested Frosst & Co. to prepare 500 mg tablets of niacin, niacinamide, and placebo. Both companies sent us their vitamins free of charge. I imagine this minor investment by these companies has been amply repaid since by the vast sales of niacin, especially for lowering cholesterol values. Our discovery that niacin lowered cholesterol levels came from these free supplies.

In our pilot studies, the compound was given to patients to determine how best to use it and how much to give for optimum results, thus to establish dose ranges. We were not concerned about toxicity because water soluble vitamins had all ready been shown to be safe, and with animal studies enormous doses were required before any toxicity could be demonstrated. With dogs, around 5 grams per kilogram of body weight would kill half the animals tested. In human terms it would mean giving 250 grams (about half a pound) to a 50 kg person. It would be impossible to consume that amount because the sheer bulk of it would cause severe nausea and vomiting long before the toxic dose could be reached. Later we found that the nauseant dose varied enormously. One of my young patients, in a fit of pique against her mother, swallowed two hundred 500 mg niacin tablets. Later on she complained her abdomen was sore. Another teenager, on her own took 50 grams per day. The highest dose I have used is 32 grams on one patient; most have taken 12 grams per day or less, and the vast majority took between 3 and 6 grams daily.

The second meeting of the Saskatchewan Committee on Schizophrenia, June 30, 1952, was held in the Medical Building, University of Saskatchewan at Saskatoon. Present were Dr C. MacArthur, Professor of Biochemistry, Dr D. E. Hutcheon, Professor of Pharmacology in the Department of Physiology, Dr V. Woodford, Professor of Biochemistry, Dr J. Lucy, psychiatrist at Saskatchewan Hospital, Weyburn, Dr H. Osmond, Clinical Superintendent of that hospital, with me as chairman. Dr Osmond reported the results of giving nicotinic acid to six patients. I added two cases from the Munro Wing, General Hospital, Regina.

Dr Osmond presented us with the following results:

෴ 1. P.B.(about age 50): Mr. B. had failed to respond to treatment at the Munro Wing and had been transferred to Weyburn. Normally this would have meant many years of treatment. His neuropsychiatrist at the Munro Wing, a distinguished former professor of neuropsychiatry in Europe, considered his diagnosis to be either Alzheimer's or catatonic schizophrenia. At Weyburn he remained quiet and passive for a few days, before suddenly becoming violently psychotic, expressing delusions he would be poisoned or killed. He was given niacinamide, 1 gram daily. In four days he was well and remained well for six weeks, at which time he was discharged.

෴ 2. D.C.(age 22): Ken was admitted in February 1952, very ill and violently psychotic. He received a series of ECT, improved for a brief period and then relapsed. He was started on insulin coma therapy and gradually became worse. He was placed in restraint. Eventually he became comatose. The senior psychiatrist concluded he was dying and so informed Dr Osmond. It was agreed his family should be notified.

However, I suggested to Humphry we should start him on both vitamin B-3 and C, as his clinical condition was desperate. Because he was in a coma and could not eat or drink, we placed a tube into his stomach and poured in 5 grams of niacin and 5 grams of ascorbic acid. That evening he came out of his coma. The next day he was able to sit up and drink. Two weeks later, on a daily dose of 5 grams of niacin plus 5 grams of ascorbic acid, he was well. His family took him home four weeks later.

I interviewed this patient in Saskatoon many years later. He had no recollection of having been in hospital. He was normal, a successful business man in his community.

☙ 3. A.L. (age 50): Mrs. L. had been admitted to hospital several times, showing both schizophrenic and manic-depressive features. She would recover temporarily after a series of ECT. She was very paranoid, convinced that everyone was listening to her and that the radio was broadcasting about her. To protect herself she began to tear out heat registers and plug up the pipes. She became a very difficult nursing problem. On 5 grams of niacin and 5 grams of ascorbic acid each day, after a few weeks she was no longer any nursing problem. When the vitamins were discontinued she relapsed, but was still better than she had been.

☙ 4. M.L. (age 20): This young woman became psychotic after childbirth. After a series of ECT her psychosis temporarily subsided. She was then given 60 insulin coma treatments. She was started on niacin and ascorbic acid. She began to improve in a week, was ready for discharge in two more weeks, and was well one month after discharge.

☙ 5. A.M.: He was admitted very disturbed and it was impossible to obtain a history. He was noisy, very hostile, and staff was very fearful of him. He was given niacin and a series of three ECT, and was well in three days.

☙ 6. T.M.: Very ill on admission, he was unkempt, dirty, masturbated openly and kept repeating, "It is too late." He had been treated in hospital one-and-one-half years before. He was started on 10 grams of niacin plus 10 grams of ascorbic acid per day; on the fourth day he was well.

I reported on two additional patients treated at the Munro Wing:

☙ 1. Mr. F. (age 39): Mr. F. had been ill three months. He was an army veteran who had survived the war well. With his psychosis he became convinced the Canadian army had plotted against him and that his neighbors were all plotting against him. He was started on niacin 1 gram per day. Ten days later he fled from hospital. At home, he told his parents he had come back to check out whether his neighbors were plotting against him. He was brought back to hospital and the niacin was increased to 2 grams per day. Several weeks later he was improved enough to be discharged. A few months later he was normal. On follow-up he remained well thereafter, in spite of going through very difficult economic problems on his farm.

2. Miss G. (age 45): When she was seventeen, Miss G. had suffered a rapid change in her personality and mood. After recovery she remained very shy. In December 1950 following an office party, she started thinking her employer loved her and planned to leave his wife, which disturbed her very much. There had been no change in her employer which could have precipitated these paranoid delusions. In April 1951 she was admitted to hospital and given nine ECT. She became well and returned to work as a senior stenographer for a very large Saskatchewan company. In December 1951, following another staff party, the same thought disorder recurred and she was again admitted. She hallucinated, was very delusional and depressed. The day she was admitted to hospital she tried twice to kill herself. She was given eight ECT and intensive psychotherapy three hours per week. She improved, but a few months after discharge had to be re-admitted on April 10, 1952.

Normally, she would then have been transferred to Saskatchewan Hospital Weyburn, but I decided to start her on niacin. I had been waiting for a patient who was clearly schizophrenic, who had not responded very well to our best treatment in 1952: ECT and psychotherapy. I started her on niacin 1 gram three times per day. One month later she was better and was discharged. She remained on the vitamin for three months thereafter and then stopped taking the pills. One month later she again relapsed. Her employer by this time was fed up with her frequent relapses and medical leaves. Her sister brought her back to hospital; again she was paranoid, hostile, and negative. This time her sister agreed to supervise her medication, and she stayed on the niacin until October 1953. She had survived another Christmas staff party without relapsing. In December 1953 her paranoid ideas reappeared. She was persuaded to start back on niacin and remained on it until 1956; this time I agreed she could discontinue. In December 1964 she was still well, free of symptoms, friendlier, and still working at her job. As far as I know, she has never relapsed.

Dr Osmond and I were very excited by these results. In the minutes of the meeting I wrote, "The number of patients treated so far does provide very exciting information, but as no well-controlled clinical trial was run the results are not entirely conclusive. These were preliminary trials in order to determine how to use these drugs. Adequately controlled trials are now planned and will be run off as quickly as possible."

Over the next two years, twenty-nine schizophrenic patients were started on niacin 3 grams per day. Most suffered from hallucinations and delusions. They were diagnosed by the treating psychiatrists, who would use ECT if necessary, using the criteria in common use in 1952. If the psychiatrist agreed and if I concurred with the diagnosis, they were given the vitamin. The patients were all evaluated by the end of 1954. They were evaluated at discharge and thereafter at three month intervals.

Improvement was evaluated by the therapist and, after discharge, by the social worker. The number evaluated toward the end of the follow-up period was less than at the onset because fewer patients had been as long in the community. One of the best markers for improvement was their ability to stay in the community. In 1952 abnormal behavior was not tolerated, especially after once having been in a psychiatric hospital, and patients would promptly be brought back to hospital by family or the police.

Over 90 percent of the twenty-nine patients given niacin with or without ECT were improved at discharge and one year later. This compares with the twenty-one patients given vitamin B-3 in the double blind experiment which followed our pilot trials, of whom around 80 percent were still well. The treatment outcome of the nine patients given placebo was the usual spontaneous recovery rate said to be characteristic of acute schizophrenia. This 29-patient pilot study foreshadowed the results we would obtain later with the 30-patient double-blind controlled experiment. See Table 1 for a summary of these results.

FIRST DOUBLE-BLIND CONTROLLED EXPERIMENT

At the second meeting of the Saskatchewan Committee on Schizophrenia Research, we had concluded that controlled studies would be required to test vitamin B-3's therapeutic potential. It was highly unlikely, although possible, that eight patients who had not responded to the only treatments then in use — psychotherapy, insulin coma or ECT — would all respond to vitamin B-3 and that no other patients would enjoy similar recoveries. With controlled studies we could test the hypothesis that these preliminary responses were chance — i.e., spurious — or that other patients would also respond. By well-controlled studies we meant that we would randomize patients into untreated or treated groups in order to compare standard treatment — ECT and psychotherapy — against ECT, psychotherapy, and vitamin B-3. My training toward my PhD in agricultural biochemistry had included courses in biostatistics. Comparison studies had become well-established in agricultural research.

TABLE 1
Comparison of Niacin Alone and Niacin
and ECT on Follow-Up State, by Months

Group	Number	Disch.	3	6	9	12	15	18
Niacin	Evaluated	17	17	16	14	11	6	4
	Improved	16	14	16	13	10	6	4
	Percentage	94	89	100	93	90	100	100
Niacin	Evaluated	19	19	10	6	6	3	3
and ECT	Improved	8	7	7	5	6	3	3
	Percentage	67	58	70	83	100	100	100
All Niacin	Evaluated	29	29	26	20	17	9	7
	Improved	24	21	23	18	16	9	7
	Percentage	83	72	88	88	95	100	100

A few months later, Dr C. Roberts, Director, Mental Health Division of the Department of Health, Ottawa, approached us. One of the drug companies from Quebec was preparing to release a nucleotide preparation as a treatment for chronic schizophrenia, based upon clinical studies conducted in one of Quebec's largest mental hospitals. A chemist had developed a yeast nucleotide fraction which he had injected into a number of patients. He reported that about 50 percent responded. However, the Department of Health did not want this product released until controlled studies had been conducted in another hospital. The company agreed to withhold release of their product until the results of these tests were available. They promised to provide material and other support. Dr Roberts could find no other hospital willing to run this experiment.

He invited Humphry Osmond and me to Ottawa, and from there drove us to Montreal. We also met Dr Bud Fisher, a virologist who had caught an infection from a virus he was researching. He nearly died and was left permanently scarred, and he was forbidden from ever doing viral research again. He became a statistician and advisor to Dr

Roberts on applications for research grants.

Dr Fisher suggested we do the research in a double-blind manner. In England this type of experiment was called "double dummy." This was the method used to test the anti-arthritis properties of corticosteroids against aspirin. We asked Dr Fisher to let us have the details of this new method, as we had not heard anything about it before.

Double-blind methodology is based upon the hypothesis that patients can respond to an inert material if they have an expectation of being helped — the placebo response. It is also based upon the idea that investigators who do not know what treatment the patient is receiving will be more free of bias in making their evaluation. Thus, the double-blind controlled experiment is supposed to guarantee: (1) that both groups being tested are approximately equal — i.e., all will be drawn from the larger population of patients with the same disease; (2) there will be no placebo effect to invalidate the results; and (3) observer bias will be minimized.

These propositions made sense to us, and we agreed to run these therapeutic trials using the nucleotide preparation and a placebo. The preparation was given by injection, as was the placebo. This was the first double-blind experiment ever carried out in psychiatry. We completed these studies in a couple of years, but found that none of the chronic patients improved, whether given placebo or active compound. Because we saw no response, the experiment was discontinued half-way through the series. We considered it unethical to continue treating patients with two different sets of inert injections. We also proved that chronic schizophrenics were not placebo responders.

Our double-blind design was developed in consultation with Dr Fisher, but tailored to our clinical needs. For example, Bud Fisher did not want us to use ECT as it would increase the difficulty in assessing the outcome. However, ECT was the only treatment which would calm an aggressive, ferocious patient. Without ECT these patients would need violent restraint in a locked room. After a series of ECT they would be calmer, more relaxed, and less depressed; there were no tranquilizers at this time. But with a truly randomized double-blind design, ECT would be given to all tested groups at about the same ratio of those who did or did not receive it. As a rule, ECT was given to more severely psychotic patients.

Having mastered the double-blind design, we decided to use it in testing the value of vitamin B-3. The first trial was conducted at the Munro Wing, the psychiatric ward of the General Hospital at Regina, Saskatchewan. It was managed by the hospital, supported by the Psychiatric Services Branch, and was under clinical control of the Psychiatric Services Branch. The clinical director reported directly to Dr G. McKerracker, as did I, as Director of Psychiatric Research.

Patients from southern Saskatchewan were admitted to the ward. They were not as sick as those sent to the mental hospital at Weyburn. The Munro Wing admitted about 45 schizophrenic patients per year, plus all other diagnostic groups, to the 39-bed ward, while about 150 per year were admitted to the 2000-bed mental hospital. Patients who did not respond in a few months were sent to the mental hospital for long-term care.

In 1952 we used the diagnostic criteria for schizophrenia proposed by Bleuler about 1900. The diagnosis was made by the treating resident in consultation with the psychiatrist in charge, neither of whom were members of the research group. All schizophrenics admitted to the ward were eligible for the vitamin study; as soon as a patient was diagnosed schizophrenia, I was informed. If the treating doctor did not wish his patient to be in the study, the patient would not be used, but this occurred rarely. The therapists used another way to keep their patients out of the study: they would diagnose them chronic anxiety or depression, thus making them ineligible. The first year of our study there was a significant decrease in the number of schizophrenic patients admitted to the ward, but in the second year the numbers went up as diagnosis could no longer be delayed. For example, one resident who had diagnosed his patient as an anxiety state, treated her with intensive psychotherapy three hours per week. There was no improvement. Several months later I interviewed her for other reasons and discovered she was having hallucinations of her sister, whom she could see sitting near the ceiling in the corner of her room. I reported this to her resident, and he promptly sent her to the mental hospital; he had no interest in giving schizophrenics psychotherapy.

After I was informed that a patient was available, I interviewed them. If I concurred with the diagnosis, they were included in the study. Today I am still convinced that every one of these patients was, in fact, schizophrenic.

Patients were assigned a number from 1 to 30 as they were admitted. They were then given a battery of physiological and psychological tests before they were started on medication. Their own doctor could use either psychotherapy or ECT, or both, for the patient, but insulin subcoma was not permitted. There were no tranquilizers at this time, so this did not complicate our studies.

We used three treatments: placebo, niacinamide, or niacin, giving patients 1 gram three times per day for thirty days. We could not use only niacin and placebo, because the niacin flush would immediately betray to staff who was taking it, but with niacinamide there was no flushing. However, we informed clinical staff that only niacin and placebo were being used. They therefore thought all patients who flushed were on niacin, and that the remainder were on placebo. In fact, half of those patients who did not flush were on niacinamide, and the other half were on placebo.

The three treatments were randomized by coin toss into

three groups. Bottles of pills were prepared for us by a drug company and were numbered from 1 to 30. The order in which the patient was diagnosed determined what they got. The code was kept by the dispensary and was not available to anyone. We had decided in advance to break the code one year after the last patient was treated and evaluated, but there were two exceptions: patients who completed the treatment and had not improved at all, or who had improved but relapsed after discharge, were exempted. Their resident could then ask for that patient's code to be broken. The resident could then, if he wished, start the patient on niacin or niacinamide, but that patient was then classed as a treatment failure. Patients were given the same battery of physiological and psychological tests after two weeks and again after four weeks when the therapeutic trial was over.

After discharge, a trained social worker followed up each patient using a standardized questionnaire. They were seen every three months until one year had passed. As the code had not been broken, the social worker was also blind.

I was not surprised by the outcome since I had all ready seen so many patients respond before this trial was started, but it was very exciting to have these positive results which proved that for the type of patients treated at the Munro Wing, we had a treatment which was more effective than placebo or ECT used alone. It also showed that the flush caused by niacin was not a factor because the results were equally good with niacinamide. With niacin we had doubled the two year recovery rate from about 35 percent to about 70 percent. See Table 2 for a summary of these results.

The results were impressive but generated a lot of ambivalence among the clinical staff. After we had all the data in and had uncovered the code, we reported the results at a clinical meeting of physicians, nurses, and social workers. My recollection is that there was no great burst of enthusiasm. I believe it was impossible for psychiatrists to believe that a vitamin could help a disease as terrifying and

TABLE 2
Summary of Thirty Day Trial, After One Year

Treatment	Number	Days In Hospital	Number On ECT	Number Sent To Weyburn	Number Well
Placebo	9	63	6	0	3
Niacin	10	60	7	1	8
Niacinamide	11	72	7	2	9

mysterious as schizophrenia, and that such a discovery could have been made at their hospital. It was simply too good to be true. In fact our boss, Dr D. G. McKerracker, concluded his remarks by saying that if what we had found was true, we would get the Nobel Prize. As soon as he said that, I developed the uneasy feeling we were heading into difficult waters. His statement may have easily meant that, since it was highly unlikely we would ever get the Nobel Prize, it was equally unlikely that what we had found was true.

Later he urged us not to publish our data, saying it was most important we be absolutely sure before we disclosed what we had discovered. We therefore decided to start a second, much larger double-blind controlled experiment, using new patients and testing 120. We called it the "120 Project."

CLINICAL STUDIES

In the meantime, our open clinical studies continued at the Munro Wing and at Weyburn. A double-blind study answers only one question: is the active compound more effective than placebo? It does not give any information about side effects, toxicity, duration of treatment required, optimum dose, changes in doses with recovery, maintenance doses, and so on.

I compared all schizophrenics who had received vitamin B-3 between 1951 and 1954, either as in-patients or out-patients, with all the other schizophrenic patients treated at the same time by placebo or by ECT, insulin sub-coma, and psychotherapy. There were 171 patients who fell into four distinct groups. They were evaluated in 1955, with results as shown in Tables 3 and 4:

- 1. Those who received vitamin B-3 in hospital and after discharge.
- 2. Those who received vitamin B-3 after discharge.
- 3. Those who received vitamin B-3 in hospital.
- 4. Those who did not receive any vitamin B-3.

TABLE 3
Effect of Treatment

Group	Number	Days In Hospital	Number On ECT	Number Sent To Mental Hospital	Number Suicide	State Well*
1	24	58	10	1	0	78
2	13	40	1	0	0	80
3	36	74	23	6	0	81
4	98	50	47	47	4	60

*This figure gives the percentage of the group who were well.

I also compared the number of re-admissions of the control (no Vitamin B-3 and the treated groups.

TABLE 4
Effect of Vitamin B-3 on Admissions

Treatment	No.	1	2	3	4	5	Days in Hosp. P/Pt.	In Hosp.
Control	98	27	11	6	2	1	319	7
Vit. B-3	73	7	1	0	0	0	234	0

At the end of our studies at the Munro Wing in 1955, we kept our conclusions low key. We wrote, "When used in adequate dosages, nicotinic acid and nicotinamide materially contributed to the recovery of schizophrenic patients."

PROJECT 120

We started this study in Regina, admitting patients from June 1953 to April 30, 1955. Then we moved to our new research area at University Hospital and began to admit patients to this study October 1955 to the end of 1958. We were not able to acquire 120 patients as it was becoming too difficult. At the Munro Wing, tranquilizers had not yet begun to play the major role they did at University Hospital. The response to vitamins was slow, and therapists were too impatient to wait for it when tranquilizers promised to be even better, much more quickly. Our design, laid down before tranquilizers were available, did not allow their use for patients entering the study. We decided to terminate the study after completing 82 patients.

The same design as in the first double-blind study was used, except that niacinamide was not included. Using only niacin and placebo simplified the design. However, the clinical staff was advised there would be a niacinamide group. They would therefore believe that half of the non-flushers were on niacinamide, when in fact they were all on placebo. This trial ran for 33 days.

If a patient failed to respond, the therapist could ask for that patient's code to be broken. He then had the option of giving the patient niacin, but, as in the previous trial, that patient was then classed as a treatment failure. The number of requests from each group was thus another measure of response. This request was made eighteen times for the placebo group, and only once for the niacin group. This difference is highly significant: Chi Square = 19. See Table 5 for the results of this trial.

TABLE 5
Comparison of Niacin and Placebo Group From
Second Double-Blind Controlled Experiment

Group	No.	Mean Age	Number Receiving	Mean Days In Hosp. ECT	Not Improved	Improved
Placebo	43	31.8	21	74	18	25
Niacin	39	30.3	15	72	31	8

FOLLOW-UP STUDIES

I had hoped to enter all patients into a new community double-blind treatment trial after discharge. They were started on 1 gram per day of either niacin or placebo. Patients who were classed as treatment failures and then placed on niacin were not included in this community study. Patients sent to the mental hospitals were also dropped from any subsequent study. Patients who remained on the double blind study were sent their tablets labeled "Treatment Tablets." In 1959 a final evaluation was made, and I personally interviewed most of the patients. After that the treatment code was broken.

The course of schizophrenia is variable, so it is difficult to quantify recovery exactly. Thus, a patient may have remained well for eleven months and been sick in the twelfth, or the patient may have been sick for six months and then well by the twelfth month. I used a patient/year index. If a patient had been well two years, he had a well patient/year index of 2. A patient was "well" when free of all signs and symptoms of illness. A patient was considered "much improved" if he still had some signs and symptoms of illness, but got on well in the community, was employed or busy at his or her usual pre-psychosis activity, and got on well with family. If the patient had signs and symptoms of illness but only got on well in two areas, he was classed as "improved." Patients were "not improved" if they were only able to stay out of hospital because of the tolerance and kindness of their families. One example of an "improved" patient would be a delusional patient who was able to get on well with family, able to do household activities, but who was not able to be involved in any community activities.

More than half the time, patients from the placebo-niacin groups were well or much improved. Only 20 percent of the placebo-placebo group were in this improved state. It was evident that niacin over the long haul after discharge, was more effective than one month of niacin in hospital. This agrees with my observations made on thousands of patients since that time: recovery on vitamin B-3 is slow but steady.

Readmission data is an excellent measure of relapse, but one must count the patients admitted, the number of re-admissions, and the duration of each readmission in days or months. In this study, 91 percent of the community years from the niacin-niacin group were free of re-admissions. The placebo-placebo group fared less well, readmitting patients 21 out of 56 community years, leaving 62 percent of the community years free of re-admissions.

The entire group on niacin were readmitted 38 times for 67 admissions, averaging 64 days per patient. The entire placebo group (or non-niacin group) were readmitted 36 times for 81 admissions averaging 147 days per patient — i.e., using niacin decreased re-admissions more than 50 percent. Out of the all-niacin group, 28 percent of patients required readmission. From the all-niacin group, 31 percent were readmitted. From the first group, for each patient relapsing there were 1.5 admissions. From the second group, each readmitted patient was readmitted 2.3 times.

If we look upon the four groups as different treatments and compare the merits of each one by the number of patients readmitted, the number of re-admissions, the number of patients well or much improved, and by the number of five-year cures, then the best treatment was niacin-niacin,

TABLE 6
Percentage of Group Re-Admissions per Year

	Years After Discharge					
	1	2	3	4	5	Total
Placebo-Placebo	40	21	40	55	50	40
Placebo-Niacin	13	25	25	30	0	20
Niacin-Placebo	36	24	17	13	41	26
Niacin-Niacin	8	12	4	6	20	10

The next table shows the impact of using niacin on admissions over the follow-up period.

TABLE 7

	Discharge	Number Admit	Admiss	In Hospital Days	Avg/Pt	Rnge
P–P	20	7	16	3318	207	7-1584
N–P	29	13	24	2875	120	7-344
P–N	8	2	6	326	54	31-123
N–N	25	5	9	925	103	23-184
N in Community	33	7	15	1251	91	
All Niacin	62	20	39	4126	106	

followed in descending order of merit by placebo-niacin, niacin-placebo, and the last, placebo-placebo. These results are shown in Tables 6, 7, and 8.

I then examined the results of the treatment of all schizophrenic patients treated by four different psychiatrists at University Hospital, Saskatoon, between October 1, 1955, and December 31, 1962, and evaluated after August 17, 1964. Psychiatrists A and C routinely would not use vitamin B-3 or reserved it only for their failures toward the end of the treatment. Psychiatrist B routinely did use vitamin B-3 and encouraged patients to stay on it after discharge. I am Psychiatrist D.

Psychiatrists A and C only used niacin on their failures, then reluctantly, and never after discharge. The main treatments they used were tranquilizers, psychotherapy, and ECT, but even so, their patients given vitamin B-3 fared better than their patients not given vitamin B-3. Psychiatrist A's vitamin patients were readmitted for an average of 80 days for the entire group, and there were none in hospital and no suicides. His non-vitamin group required 113 days per day in

TABLE 8
Effect of Niacin on Number of Re-Admissions

Treatment	No.	Re-Admitted	Re-Admissions	Ttl Yrs.	Dys P/Pt	Dys /Adm
Niacin-Niacin	49	12	19	7.5	56	147
Niacin-Placebo	65	21	38	14.9	84	155
Placebo-Niacin	22	5	19	1.2	20	184
Placebo-Placebo	117	36	81	47.1	147	209
All Niacin	136	38	67	23.8	64	139

re-admissions, 8 were in hospital, and 3 had killed themselves.

Psychiatrist C had very similar results. From the "Vitamin" group they required 49 days per patient re-admissions (for the entire group), and one was in hospital. There were no suicides. Of the "Other Treatment" group, 6 were in hospital and 2 had killed themselves.

Psychiatrist B used vitamin B-3 but not with the same interest that I had. I encouraged my patients both in hospital and outside hospital to carry on as long as possible. His patients needed only 44 days per patient for the entire group, and one was in hospital. His "Other Treatment" group needed 70 days in hospital, and none were in. There were no suicides from either group.

My vitamin group needed 61 days in hospital per patient (entire group of 56), and one was in hospital. My smaller "Others" group needed 217 days, and one was in hospital.

The 232 "Other" group needed 35,032 days, or 96 years in hospital over a six-year period, or 16 admissions per year. The 128 "Vitamin" group needed 7,424 days, or 20 years, in hospital, i.e., 3.3 years of admissions per year. If the Other group had been given vitamins, they would have required 13,456 days, or 37 years, a saving of 59 patient years, or 9.8 patient years per year. At current costs of about $1000 per day or $365,000 per patient year, this equals $357,700 per year. From this ward of 37 beds, only 27 would have been required. Extrapolating to other psychiatric wards, this suggests one could decrease the bed capacity by one-third, a significant saving of money. See Tables 9 and 10 for a summary of these results.

CHRONIC PATIENTS

The majority of patients admitted to University Hospital were admitted for the first time to any ward. Failures

TABLE 9
Treatment Results
Psychiatrist A

Year Treated	N	Re-Admt.	N Re-Admss.	N Dys Admt.	Days P/Pt.	N in Hsp. 08/17/64	N. Suicide
On Niacin							
1956-57	8	1	2	98	12	0	0
58	2	0	0	0	0	0	0
59	2	1	2	50	25	0	0
60	6	4	9	843	140	0	0
61	1	0	0	0	0	0	0
62	3	1	1	760	253	0	0
Total	22	7	14	1751	80	0	0
Other Treatment–No Niacin							
1956-57	34	18	56	3916	115	1	0
58	18	14	50	3999	222	0	1
59	13	7	16	589	46	1	1
60	23	13	26	1411	61	1	1
61	20	10	21	2233	112	2	0
62	29	14	33	3290	114	3	0
Total	137	76	202	15438	113	8	3

Year Treated	N	Re-Admt.	N Re-Admss.	N Dys Admt.	Days P/Pt.	N in Hsp. 08/17/64	N. Suicide
Psychiatrist B								
On Niacin								
1956-57	5	2	4	229	46	0	0
58	6	1	2	256	43	0	0
59	8	2	6	174	22	0	0
60	9	2	8	525	58	0	0
61	10	5	12	480	48	0	0
Total	38	12	32	1664	44	0	0
Other Treatment								
1956-57	4	2	5	607	152	0	0
58	1	1	1	202	202	0	0
59	3	2	5	238	79	0	0
60	5	1	2	90	18	0	0
61	3	2	2	154	51	0	0
62	4	2	2	107	27	0	0
Total	20	10	17	1398	70	0	0

Year Treated	N	Re-Admt.	N Re-Admss.	N Dys Admt.	Days P/Pt.	N in Hsp. 08/17/64	N. Suicide
Psychiatrist C
On Niacin
1956-57	4	2	3	223	56	0	0
58	3	2	4	197	66	1	0
59	4	1	2	33	8	0	0
61	1	1	5	133	133	0	0
Total	12	6	14	586	49	1	0
Other Treatment
1956-57	22	16	33	7880	358	1	0
58	10	7	29	3664	366	3	0
59	7	2	5	321	46	0	2
60	14	8	20	2792	200	1	0
61	9	6	16	1659	184	1	0
62	4	3	7	517	129	0	0
Total	66	42	110	16833	255	6	2

FOLLOW-UP STUDIES 61

Psychiatrist D

Year Treated	N	Re-Admt.	N Re-Admss.	N Dys Admt.	Days P/Pt.	N in Hsp. 08/17/64	N. Suicide
\multicolumn{8}{c}{On Niacin — First Admissions}						
1956-57	19	9	16	2117	111	1	0
58	9	5	9	363	40	0	0
59	4	1	1	4	1	0	0
60	9	3	3	701	78	0	0
61	4	1	1	42	11	0	0
62	11	6	8	194	18	0	0
Total	56	25	38	3421	61	1	0
\multicolumn{8}{c}{Chronic Patients}						
1956-57	16	12	25	3428	214	1	0
58	5	5	9	3004	600	1	0
59	4	3	7	1873	468	1	0
60	3	2	4	416	139	0	0
61/62	7	1	6	206	29	0	0
Total	35	23	51	8927	255	3	0
\multicolumn{8}{c}{Other Treatment}						
	9	6	21	1304	217	1	0

TABLE 10
Summary of all Four Psychiatrists

Psych.	N	N Re-Admt.	N Re-Admss.	N Dys Admt.	Days P/Pt.	N in Hsp. 08/17/64	N. Suicide
On Niacin							
A	22	7	14	1751	80	0	0
B	38	12	32	1664	44	0	0
C	12	6	14	586	49	1	0
D	56	25	38	3421	61	1	0
Total	128	50	98	7422	58	2	0
No Niacin							
A	137	76	202	15438	113	8	3
B	20	10	17	1398	70	0	0
C	66	42	110	16833	255	6	2
D	9	6	21	1304	217	1	0
Total	232	134	350	34973	151	15	5
Mental Hosp. Group	114	43	119	19518	171	14	1
All No Niacin	346	177	469	54491	157	2	0

from previous treatment programs were not admitted to the services of other psychiatrists. Because I was interested in chronic schizophrenia, I did admit failures from my treatment as well as failures from other programs. These re-admissions are chronic patients.

Chronic patients did not respond as well as acute patients. My chronic group was admitted in order to study the long-term use of vitamin B-3 for chronics. They fared least well of all the treated patients, but they were better off than were other treated patients. As the treatment period passed the seven-year mark, I noted with some surprise that many of these chronic patients began to recover. See Tables 11 and 12 for a summary of the results of this study.

Chronic schizophrenic patients given vitamin B-3 for short periods of time, i.e., up to a year, did not respond to treatment. This had always puzzled me, but does not any more. Once I had accepted the concept of syndromes, it began to make sense. Vitamin B-3 would be most useful for patients whose schizophrenia arose from a dependency on vitamins. Patients who are ill primarily because they are suffering from one or more food allergies, such as dairy products or wheat, would be a lot less responsive. The cerebral allergic syndrome is a schizophrenic reaction to chronic use of these foods. Vitamin B-3 does have anti-allergic properties: niacin decreases histamine levels by markedly lowering concentration from its storage sites. The evidence is persuasive; the first dose of niacin causes the most intense flush or vasodilation. Gradually, over days or weeks, this reaction becomes less intense, until there is only a very slight reaction or none at all. If niacin is not taken for a few days, patients will again experience some flushing.

About 1970 I began to examine schizophrenic patients for food allergies by fasting patients 4 to 5 days. If allergies were present, the patient would be much better at the end of the fast. Then individual foods were reintroduced and the patient's reaction observed; the foods which caused a relapse would be the ones to which that

TABLE 11
Acute and Chronic Schizophrenic Patients and Their Response to Treatment
Psychiatrist D

	N Re-Admt.	N Readmitted	Niacin (D) N Readmissions	Mean Days	N In	Suicides
Acute	56	25	38	61	1	0
Chronic	35	23	51	255	3	0
Others	9	6	21	217	1	0

All Psychiatrists

		N	N Readmitted	N Readmissions
Acute	NAC	113	82	54
	Other	150	206	107
Chronic	NAC	50	67	206
	Other	58	117	297

patient was allergic, and these foods would be eliminated from the diet thereafter.

Before 1970 I routinely gave my chronic patients 12 grams of niacin or more per day. They improved, but often did not recover. After they went onto the allergy-free diet, within a few days or weeks they were no longer able to tolerate the same dose of niacin, which had to be quickly reduced to 3 to 6 grams daily. This happened so often I became convinced it was a real phenomenon. Niacin did counteract some of the allergic reactions to these foods.

I suspect niacin acts as an anti-allergen because it does lower histamine levels. It is therefore therapeutic, but it does not act very quickly. Many years may be required before chronic patients respond, but psychiatrists in hospitals only see patients for short periods. The usual therapeutic trials will be of no value for chronic patients. They must be treated for many years — as they are today with

TABLE 12

Psychiatrist	Treatment	N	Readmitted	Readmissions	Mean Days	N In	N Suicide
*A	NAC	22	7 32%	14	80	0	0
	Other	137	76 55%	202	113	8	3
B	NAC	38	12 32%	32	44	0	0
	Other	20	10 50%	17	70	0	0
*C	NAC	12	6 50%	14	49	1	0
	Other	66	42 64%	110	255	6	2
D	NAC	56	25 45%	38	61	1	0
	Other	9	6 67%	21	217	1	0
Mental Hospital	Other	114	43	119	171	14	1

*Psychiatrist A & C only used niacin for treatment of failures.

	All Niacin	128	50 39%	98	58	2	0
	All Other	232	134 58%	350	151	15	5
	Mental Hosp.	114	43 38%	119	171	14	1

tranquilizers. An entire system has been developed to keep patients on tranquilizers including psychiatrists, general practitioners, home nurses who will deliver them to patients and inject them, hospital parenteral centers, financial relief, and even legal sanctions. None of these systems is in place for the use of nutrition and vitamins. In fact, the system is used to prevent patients following such a program.

An example of a recovery is the case of Pauline. She was born in 1927 and was admitted to the Munro Wing October 5, 1953. At age 19, a voice told her she was pregnant, and since she had not had relations, she considered this a miracle. Later, when symptoms of pregnancy did not develop, she concluded she was not pregnant. Two years later another voice told her she had a powerful body odor. One year after that, Satan began regularly to insult her; this continued for four years. Before her admission to hospital, a different voice again told her she was pregnant and that she was the bride of Christ. She was by this time having frequent visual and auditory hallucinations of Christ and Satan. She was convinced Christ would come from heaven on a chariot and would transport her bodily back with him. In order to prepare for this, she gave up her job and spent most of her time studying the Bible. Her mother was able to tolerate her behavior because she herself as a young woman had gone through a brief psychosis.

There was no question about her diagnosis, which was based upon her hallucinations, thought disorder, flat mood, and behavior consistent with her delusions. However, Pauline was convinced there was nothing wrong with her and refused to take any medication. I persuaded her to try niacin, which I suggested would make her physically stronger and would not stop her religious visitations. I discharged her from hospital November 21, 1953.

After that her improvement was slow but steady. On January 2, 1954, she reported Satan was not as troublesome. Now and then she wished she were normal. By October 13,

1954, she planned to go back to work. June 6, 1955, she was much better; she still suffered from hallucinations but they no longer preoccupied her. May 11, 1957, she was at ease, cheerful. She taught Sunday school, helped her mother, but on occasion did hear voices. She had decreased her niacin to 1 gram daily. February 17, 1958, she was employed full-time. July 25, 1960, she wrote, "I am getting along fine and have really been keeping busy. This winter I took a course in typing, and with teaching Sunday school and all the other activities, I did not have too much time for other things, but now that summer is here, I have been spending more time going to the beach and picnic with friends."

On October 1, 1963, she wrote, "I am employed as an office clerk for a company. My work consists of filing, blueprinting, looking after the mail and a considerable amount of bookkeeping. I am also taking advanced typing and second year bookkeeping at night school." She was now normal, having met my four criteria; i.e., no signs or symptoms, getting on well with family and the community, and working full-time (paying taxes).

Over the early years I accumulated 32 chronic patients who had failed to improve even after two years of treatment. Of these, 19 did not take any vitamin B-3 once they had shown they were not responding, but 13 were maintained on niacin. Seven went to mental hospital after failing to respond to niacin, but after discharge were started on it again.

Both groups were equivalent before niacin was started and all were treatment failures for many years. There was no way anyone could have predicted which ones would have responded. There was every likelihood none would respond. The continuous niacin group were probably sicker and had been in hospital longer (552 days compared to 280 days). The group not on niacin were more often in hospital, under less pressure from the community, and were under much more psychiatric supervision. They all, or almost all, were on tranquilizers. See Tables 13, 14, and 15 for these results.

TABLE 13

Group	N Mean	Before Niacin N. Admit. Mean	Days in Hosp. Mean	After Niacin N. Admit. Mean	Days in Hosp. Mean	Present State W M1	1 Not
No NAC	19	1.3	280	3.1	691	5	13 1 died
On NAC	13	1	552	1.4	79	12	1

TABLE 14
Proportion of Time in Hospital — Chronic Schizophrenics
Years

Group	N	1956-57 Days (%)	58-59 Days (%)	60-61 Days (%)	62-63 Days (%)	1964 Days (%)
Continuous Niacin	13	864 (10.0)	686 (7.2)	516 (5.4)	447 (4.7)	96 (2.0)
Not on Niacin	19	2252 (25.0)	4178 (30.0)	3891 (28.0)	3772 (27.0)	1728 (25.0)

TABLE 15

	Total Days in Group Period	First Half Days in % Follow-up	Second Half Days in %
On NAC	3799	7538 35%	6.5%
Not on NAC	3740	8527 24%	34%

As a result of this data, I concluded in 1966 that nicotinic acid or nicotinamide should be given to every schizophrenic patient. No patient should be considered a failure until he has been on 3 grams per day for at least five years. They should also be given ECT, tranquilizers, and other drugs which will make life more tolerable for them while they are recovering. If they do not recover on this regimen, they will at least not become chronic, and whenever more effective treatments are developed, they will be in a position to take advantage of them. The vitamin will also protect them against tranquilizer toxicity since smaller doses will be just as effective.

I find it very useful to study the effect of time on a phenomenon. It is possible, although highly unlikely, that niacin worked thirty years ago due to a number of factors of which I was unaware, that these factors are different today, and that niacin would be less effective now, thirty years later. My data shows this is not true and that patients today do as well as they did several decades ago. The following case is one of my recent chronic patients who in December 1990 turned the corner and began to show major improvement. The main difference is that he is on tranquilizers as well, whereas most of my early patients in the chronic study were not.

Allan was born in 1940, and first came to see me in 1984. He told me he had been in a car accident in 1969, was unconscious for an hour, needed surgery to decompress his brain, but did recover. In 1972 he began to hear a voice, the voice of a man who lived in the same apartment building. This voice gave him advice, but also made him hurt himself. In 1981 he sought help because he could not sleep. He was given various tranquilizers, which solved his insomnia, but did nothing to this voice.

On March 5, 1984, he was admitted to a Health Sciences Center until April 16th, when his brother took him home. Later he was referred to me. He described the voice and was convinced it was from a man who had a voice machine, which projected the voice into his head. He experienced some thought blocking, and both his memory and concentration were impaired. He was very discouraged and depressed.

I started him on niacin 3 grams per day. One month later he refused to go into hospital. By September 1984 he had found a place to live in a Salvation Army group home, and they monitored his medication. January 1985 the voice was the same but he had more energy. He was still depressed. By August 1985 he was obviously better, and had more energy. In March 1986 he fell in the bathroom and required several days in hospital. The treating physician, not his G.P., stopped the niacin. In April I discovered this and he was placed back on it. He was also started on parenteral Fluanxol. By June 1987 the dose of Fluanxol was reduced to 20 mg i.m. every two weeks. August 1987 the voice was the same, but he felt better and was able to smile. He even asked me about my health. August 4, 1988, I started him on Anafranil 75 mg at bedtime. By May 1989 he found the voice less troublesome and had discovered the voice moderated when he walked. March 1990 the voice was still present but less troublesome, and his mood was good. December 1990 there was a marked improvement: he felt good, smiled, and responded appropriately. The voice was still there but he was not as fixed about the cause of it, and appeared to be more willing to accept it as a symptom of his schizophrenia.

RESULTS AFTER DISCHARGE

Patients treated with vitamin B-3 always fared better after discharge, and this was clearly related to the duration of treatment. Patients who took the vitamin continuously, as a group were healthier than patients who took it for only short periods. This finding was independent of the other treatments used such as ECT, tranquilizers, and psychotherapy, or the place where the treatment occurred. It was also independent of the orientation of the psychiatrist in charge. The most and least enthusiastic psychiatrists' patients on vitamin B-3 did better than other patients who received only placebo or other treatment. These conclusions are based upon our double-blind and clinical research studies using evaluation of mental state and also harder data such as being in hospital at evaluation, number of days in hospital, number of re-admissions, and number of suicides. The data can be summarized as follows:

From Munro Wing, Regina:

∾ 1. From the double-blind controlled experiment at two-year follow-up, 3 out of 9 on placebo were well, compared to 17 out of 21 on vitamin B-3.

∾ 2. From other clinical studies with 98 patients given vitamin B-3, there were 47 admissions averaging 319 days per patient. From 73 patients receiving other treatment only (mostly ECT and psychotherapy), there were 8 admissions averaging 234 days in hospital per patient. From this latter group there were 4 suicides.

From University Hospital:

∾ 1. From the second double-blind controlled experiment, out of 20 patients on other treatment (ECT), 3 were well five years later. But out of 62 given vitamin B-3 (with or without other treatment — ECT), 19 were well five years later.

∾ 2. From clinical studies of all patients, out of 128 given vitamin B-3, 50 were readmitted for 98 admissions totalling 7422 days (20 years); 2 were in hospital and there were no suicides. From 232 given other treatment (ECT and tranquilizers), there were 134 patients admitted for 350 admissions totalling 34,973 days (96 years); 15 patients were in hospital and 5 committed suicide. From 114 patients treated at the Saskatchewan Hospital, North Battleford, 43 patients were admitted for 119 admissions, totalling 19,518 days (53 years); 14 were in hospital and 1 killed himself. Combining all the non-vitamin groups there were 346 patients with 177 being readmitted for 469 admissions for a total of 54,491 days (149 years), 29 were in hospital and 6 committed suicide.

☙ 3. Of chronic failures, patients who had failed to respond to any treatment for at least two years, 19 were followed until 1964. About 25 percent of this group were in hospital at any time throughout this follow-up period. Thirteen were maintained on vitamin B-3 or were restarted after a period of other treatment only. With this group, the proportion of time spent in hospital decreased from 10 percent in 1956-57 to 2 percent in 1964 with a steady decrease each two years. Dividing the follow-up period into first and second half, the vitamin B-3 group decreased total days in hospital from 35 percent to 6.5 percent. In sharp contrast, the other treatment group increased total days in hospital from 24 to 34 percent.

NORTH BATTLEFORD INDEPENDENT STUDY

The data presented showed that vitamin B-3 is therapeutic for schizophrenic patients, overriding the effect of other treatment, the therapist, and the place where treatment was given. A study by Dr R. Denson on patients treated at a mental hospital confirmed this conclusion.

Dr Denson was a resident in psychiatry at Saskatchewan Hospital, North Battleford. He approached me and stated he would like to do a controlled study, as he was very skeptical vitamin B-3 had any useful therapeutic effect. Unlike most psychiatrists, his skepticism spurred him to action. I concluded he really wanted to show that the vitamin had no effect. Most psychiatrists "knew" it had no effect and did not need to explore any further.

I was pleased with his initiative and offered to help. I arranged to provide him with coded medication (vitamin B-3 and placebo), which was dispensed from the University Hospital dispensary. The code was kept by Professor J.

Summers, head of the dispensary. After the study was completed, we ran into a major problem that this study would remain forever blind, as Professor Summers was unable to find the code until some time later.

Dr Denson reported he had decided to use niacinamide because it did not cause a flush and could remain blind. Patients were new admissions or re-admissions, or returning from trial leave, and only patients who needed ECT using clinical criteria were accepted. ECT was routinely given to patients who were more ill, ill longer, and who had failed to respond to other standard treatments. Patients were selected over one year. From this cohort, 17 patients made up Group (a), and 19 went into the other group, Group (b). The two groups represented one-third of all male schizophrenic patients admitted that year. ECT and tablets were started about two weeks after admission. Any patient who was discharged from hospital before the end of the treatment period was given follow-up medication. Patients who were readmitted were not given anymore of the coded tablets, and they then received standard treatment only. The study ran from May 1959 to April 1961. Patients were also given tranquilizers as indicated. The trial run was 35 days.

Group (a), given niacinamide, were in hospital on average 106 days. The average for Group (b) on placebo was 178 days. This difference was significant. Chi Square, a measure of statistical significance, was 5.67— i.e., at a probability level of between 5 and 1 percent. Another measure used was the ratio of patients in and out of hospital. From the niacinamide group, 1 was in hospital and 16 remained in the community. From the placebo group, 8 were in hospital and 11 in the community. This was also significant at the same level.

During the first year following entry into the study, the 17 niacinamide group patients spent 1810 days in hospital, while the 19 placebo group patients spent 3373 days in hospital. (If all the patients admitted that year had been given niacinamide, they would have been in hospital 12,776 days [35 years] instead of 21,303 days [58 years] for the placebo control. This is based on about 120 admissions that year.)

Dr Denson's final conclusions were brief: patients on niacinamide spent 10 weeks less in hospital the year following entry into the study; and these results were statistically significant at a 5 percent level. He could also have pointed out the significant saving in costs: the saving of 33 patient-years in hospital out of a group of 17 patients is substantial.

This was a prospective double-blind controlled experiment which met all the criteria for clinical experiments then and now. Dr Denson practiced child psychiatry. In spite of his very good study and the excellent therapeutic response, he did not become a proponent of vitamin B-3 therapy. I can understand this, for tranquilizers had swept the psychiatric field and psychiatry became violently opposed to any therapy which supported a biochemical view of schizophrenia. Tranquilizers were considered better sedatives and therefore did not violate the well-entrenched psychosocial view of schizophrenia. Had Dr Denson reported a similar study with tranquilizers, he would have become a leader in Canadian psychiatric research — he would have been avant garde. I doubt his paper hurt his reputation since most psychiatrists remained unaware of it, even after it had been published.

SCHIZOPHRENIA AND SUICIDE

Dr Osmond and I examined the effects of treatment on suicide many years ago. Dr Nolan D. C. Lewis pointed out that suicide occurred very frequently among schizophrenics, and that this had been almost totally ignored by psychiatric textbooks.

We became aware of the importance of suicide in schizophrenia by its absence from our group treated with vitamin B-3. This was unexpected and aroused our interest, and we began systematic studies of the suicides among schizophrenics on vitamins and among schizophrenics treated with other modalities. Out of 450 patients not given vitamin B-3, 9 killed themselves over a period of 7 years. The suicide rate was about 280 per 100,000 per year. During that same period the overall rate in Saskatchewan was 9 per 100,000; i.e., about one-quarter of the suicides in Saskatchewan were schizophrenic. In our paper we reviewed the rates found by other investigators, who also found a high rate. By combining all the data from the literature and our own, the total rate was 220 per 100,000; i.e., about 20 times normal. We also reviewed 242 patients who in 1966 had been on niacin; there were no suicides.

RECOVERY

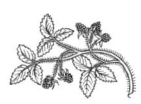

Diagnosis

The Hoffer-Osmond Diagnostic (HOD) Test

The Kryptopyrroluria (Mauve Factor) Test

Schizophrenic Syndromes

Cerebral Allergies
Vitamin Deficiencies
Vitamin B-3 Dependency
Mineral Deficiency Mineral Toxicity
The Hallucinogens

Treatment

Diet
Vitamin Supplements
Mineral Supplements
Amino Acid Supplements
Essential Fatty Acids
Electroconvulsive Treatment (ECT)
Drugs
Psychiatric Treatment

Vitamin B-3 and Mentally Disturbed Children

DIAGNOSIS

The full-blown schizophrenic syndrome is not difficult to diagnose. In fact, in most cases the problem is recognized by relatives and friends long before patients are seen by their doctors. The hallmark is unacceptable behavior, mainly because it is out of character for the person or is unpredictable. Schizophrenia is characterized by changes in perception, such as illusions and hallucinations (in severe cases, voices and visions), combined with thought disorder, which may include believing the perceptual symptoms are real, and not symptoms. Common schizophrenic thought changes are delusions, paranoid ideas, difficulty in thinking, and memory disturbance. Very often there are associated mood changes, usually depression. Schizophrenic behavior is created as a result of these perceptual changes coupled with a belief they are real. Dr Osmond and I described this in *How To Live with Schizophrenia* (1966) and I did so again in *Common Questions about Schizophrenia and Their Answers* (1988).

The onset of schizophrenia may be very rapid, although it is usually gradual. Between this onset and its full development, there is a vague set of signs and symptoms which puzzle relatives and friends, even the physicians called upon to treat them. The perceptual symptoms are usually subtle, more illusion than hallucination, and thought disorder may be minimal, suppressed by the patient. The main symptoms are changes in mood, usually some combination of anxiety, depression, and fatigue. Unless physicians ask the right questions, patients will receive a variety of non-schizophrenic diagnoses, including depression, anxiety, personality disorder, adolescent problems, etc. Only later on, as the disease progresses relentlessly, will the real diagnosis become evident. In medicine, treatment is usually most effective the earlier in the disease process it is begun; this is equally true for the schizophrenias. Response to treatment started sometime between the onset of the disease and the time it is easily recognizable as schizophrenia is usually very rapid and dramatic.

During our research with vitamin B-3 and schizophrenia, we developed two tests to aid early diagnosis: a psychological test we called the Hoffer-Osmond Diagnostic (HOD) test, and a laboratory urine test for kryptopyrrole or the mauve factor. Both pick up the early manifestations of disease when vitamin B-3 therapy is most effective. Both tests relate to each other.

The Hoffer-Osmond Diagnostic Test

Our research with schizophrenia beginning in 1952 convinced us that we had to know what our patients were experiencing in order to diagnose correctly and to understand how best to deal with them clinically. We could get this information by spending a lot of time with patients in order to question every possible perceptual change, but this would be very time-consuming and would tire them. It occurred to us that we could get at this information much more accurately and quickly by developing a set of questions to which patients could reply with a simple yes or no. General practitioners who have diagnosed schizophrenia very early on using the HOD test as an aid to diagnosis have been astonished with the rapid responses they have seen in their patients. Before these patients had been tested they were very difficult, with a lot of anxiety and depression and other vague complaints. They had not responded to the usual anti-anxiety or anti-depressant medication.

The questions were placed on cards, one question per card, and each card was numbered, beginning with 1. Patients were given these cards in random order and asked to sort them into True or False categories. Only statements which they were certain were True were accepted; the rest were considered False. All the cards said to be True were recorded on special scoring sheets.

From these True responses we prepared 145 questions. They covered all perceptual areas such as visual, auditory, tactile, taste, smell, and time. There were also questions which dealt with thinking and mood. Questions were phrased so that normal people would place most in the False category, whereas schizophrenics would place many in the True category. We then gave the test to hundreds of subjects: to schizophrenics — acute and chronic, sick, better, or well; to non-schizophrenics such as anxiety states, depressions, and personality disorders; to seniles, subjects after LSD, patients under physical stress, and to healthy people. We then compared the way each question was treated by groups; i.e., if a question was said to be True by a large proportion of schizophrenics and only very few normals, we assigned that card a special score. We scored each patient by giving each card one point if placed in the True box, and 5 points if it was a special question. We were not surprised to find that schizophrenics scored very high and normal subjects very low. We also found that one-quarter of the non-schizophrenic patients also had high scores as if they had schizophrenia; i.e., they had a large number of perceptual changes as do schizophrenics.

The HOD Test is comprised of 145 True/False questions that range from simple questions like "Most people hate me" through more complex questions like "A chair is like a table because they are usually together rather than because they both have legs" to questions like "Water now has many funny tastes." Here is a random list of other questions:

47. Some foods which never tasted funny before do now.
66. My mind is racing away with me.
81. People are watching me.
35. I have often felt that there was another voice in my head.
127. The world has become timeless for me.
17. Now and then when I look in the mirror my face changes and seems different.

90. An orange is like a banana because they both have skins rather than because they are fruit.
124. My bones often feel soft.
136. People interfere with my mind to harm me.
129. Other people smell strange.
26. I often see sparks or spots of light floating before me.
142. More people admire me now than ever before.
87. A dress is like a glove because they are articles of clothing rather than because they are worn by women.
145. I am not sure who I am.

For a full set of questions, see Appendix 1: HOD Test Questionnaire. The HOD Test is also available as a computer program and on the world wide web (www.softtac@islandnet.com).

In 1950, I observed that psychiatric diagnosis was not very stable. Patients received different diagnoses on subsequent relapses and admissions. To examine the stability of diagnosis with time, I examined the clinical records of all patients admitted more than once to the Munro Wing, between January 1, 1950 and December 31, 1954. On this ward, staff were reluctant to diagnose schizophrenia and rarely did so without clear evidence of hallucinations, delusions, catatonia, withdrawal, and other florid symptoms. The changes in diagnoses over this five year period are shown in Table 16.

TABLE 16
Changes in Diagnosis from First Admission to Re-Admission

Original Diagnosis	Final Diagnosis			
	Neuroses	Manic-Depression	Depression	Schizophrenia
Neuroses	101	9	3	20
Manic-Depression	2	21	0	1
Depression	6	3	9	2
Schizophrenia	1	1	1	48

Schizophrenia remained the most stable diagnosis. Only 3 out of 51 were re-diagnosed. Manic-depressive psychosis, now called bipolar, was almost as stable. Neuroses — i.e., the various diagnoses excluding schizophrenia and manic-depression — were the least stable. Out of 123 patients, 20 became (were re-diagnosed) schizophrenia, and 12 were re-diagnosed depression. In other words, these non-psychotics are more commonly re-diagnosed psychotic; conversely, psychotics are seldom re-diagnosed non-psychotic. I did this study 40 years ago, but from the patients I have seen over the years, it is clear the same trend exists today. The only major change is that many patients with mood swings, with or without perceptual changes or thought disorder, are diagnosed bipolar and given lithium; a response to lithium is considered by many to confirm this diagnosis. On this basis, I have suggested a simple diagnostic system. I would divide psychiatric diseases as follows:

A. Perceptual disorders
B. Thinking disorders
C. Mood disorders
D. Behavioral disorders

Group A would include the schizophrenias, some learning disorders, and some toxic psychoses. Group B would include the schizophrenias and senile disorders. Group C would include depressions, manic-depressives, and anxiety states. Group D would include all behavioral disorders. I have developed these diagnostic procedures in my book *Dr Hoffer's A,B,C of Natural Nutrition for Children with Learning Disabilities, Behavioral Disorders, and Brain Dysfunctions.*

The non-psychotic patients later diagnosed clearly schizophrenic are, according to N.D.C. Lewis and Z.A. Pietrowski, missed schizophrenics who would have been diagnosed correctly had attention been paid to their perceptual symptoms. The HOD test helps pick out the non-psychotics who will later be recognized as schizophrenic. If treatment is started before psychosis sets in, they will respond more rapidly to vitamin B-3 treatment.

Here is an example of the efficacy of the HOD test. This young patient became schizophrenic in the mid-1950s. He was treated at University Hospital, Saskatoon, with placebo, as part of our second double-blind controlled experiment. He did not respond. His treatment code was broken and he was started on niacin, 3 grams daily, plus a brief series of ECT. He recovered. Later he completed his degree and, following that, enrolled in a medical college. As I was supplying him with the vitamin from our research supply, I kept in contact with him. I advised him to stay on the niacin for five years, after which he discontinued it. About five years later, while at medical college, he again came to see me, to tell me he was not feeling well. I had him do the Hoffer-Osmond Diagnostic (HOD) Test which showed very high perceptual scores, indicating that he was suffering from many perceptual illusions. I recommended he resume his niacin. He was so desperate to get well quickly, he took 6 grams per day instead of 3, and one week later he was well again. His HOD scores returned to normal. He has remained well since that time and is practicing medicine. Had I waited for him to again suffer hallucinations, it would have required much more intense treatment, probably in hospital, and he would have lost that year of medical school.

The Kryptopyrroluria (Mauve Factor) Test

In 1960 it occurred to me that we could discover the biochemical problem in schizophrenia by using the LSD experience as a model. LSD might induce biochemical changes similar or identical to those in the schizophrenias, in the same way as it produced a model of the clinical experience. My idea was to collect samples of urine from our alcoholic patients given therapeutic LSD. If LSD could induce a similar change, a new compound or compounds not present in the urine before LSD was given might appear afterward.

We were lucky because the first alcoholic patient tested showed a characteristic mauve staining spot on the paper chromatogram after developing the paper strip with Ehrlich's reagent. See Appendix 2: Kryptopyrroluria Test Procedure for this methodology. This mauve spot was not present in the urine before LSD was given. Later we discovered LSD did not induce this material in everyone.

Once we had examined the properties of the mauve spot, we began to examine the urine of schizophrenic patients and, to our surprise, found exactly the same compound in their urine. I was surprised because I had not expected it would be so simple. Fortunately, we had a chronic female patient on our ward who excreted huge amounts of this compound, which we called "mauve factor." Later we showed it was not LSD itself or a breakdown fraction of LSD. It was identified as kryptopyrrole (KP). Many years later, after we had examined urine from thousands of patients at our four research centers, we found it was present in different psychiatric groups as follows:

Acute schizophrenics	75%
Chronic schizophrenics	50%
All non-psychotics	25%
Physically ill patients	5%
Normal subjects	0
Recovered schizophrenics	0

We could discover how many patients with schizophrenia excreted KP, but we had to show whether non-schizophrenics with KP resembled schizophrenics more than they did non-schizophrenics without KP. If they did, we could then assume that patients with KP were in fact schizophrenics. To study this, we compared large numbers of patients using clinical descriptions (diagnoses) and the HOD test. We concluded that patients who excreted KP (the mauve factor) were similar and called them "malvarians." But after the mauve factor was identified we dropped the term and used Carl Pfeiffer's more appropriate word, kryptopyrroluria, or pyrroluria, for the same group. Later, Dr Pfeiffer established pyrroluria as a schizophrenic syndrome.

In a 1963 study we compared 75 patients without malvaria to 104 patients with malvaria. The malvarians were 104 consecutive patients tested routinely over a two-year period. The non-malvarians were tested the same way. The only differences between the groups before testing were the sex ratio and the number of people who were single. The malvarian group contained more males than females, while the other group had the reverse ratio. Malvarians were more often single, and the non-malvarians were most often married. Test results are shown in Table 17.

The urine test divided 179 patients into 2 groups. A higher proportion of the malvarian group suffered from perceptual symptoms, thought disorder, and inappropriate behavior. These symptoms occurred in only 5 percent of the non-malvarians. Only in the proportion suffering from depression were they the same. Psychiatrists would have no difficulty identifying which group most closely represented schizophrenia.

On the HOD scores the malvarians had mean scores identical to schizophrenic scores, and non-malvarian scores were identical to non-schizophrenic scores. It was obvious to us that malvarians were, in fact, undiagnosed schizophrenics. If all the malvarian non-schizophrenics had been examined for perceptual changes, and had their psychiatrists taken these changes as indicators, they would have been diagnosed schizophrenia. However, their psychiatrists had no interest in our research and never asked me to divulge to them what their patients' HOD scores were.

From this data we concluded that vitamin B-3 would

TABLE 17

Clinical Description and HOD Scores

	Malvarian	Non-Malvarian
Clinical Symptom Present		
Perception	About 50%	7%
Thought	60%	4%
Mood — Inappropriate	50%	10%
Depressed	66%	66%
Activity	30%	6%
HOD Scores		
Perception	10	4
Thought	4	2.1
Mood	8	5.5
Total Score	55	26

	Schizophrenic	Non-Schizophrenic
HOD Scores		
Perception	11.9	3.4
Thought	4.0	1.5
Mood	7.1	7.8
Total Score	57	24

be therapeutic for malvarians no matter what their clinical diagnosis was, since they were most likely early or more subtle schizophrenics who hid their symptoms more successfully. They probably would respond even better, as do all diseases, if treated early.

We tested this idea and found that, in fact, vitamin B-3 was very helpful, and that this was the case regardless of their diagnosis. For example, D.S., age 31, was admitted April 21, 1960, with severe anxiety. From age 16 he drank heavily to cover his fears and inability to get along with his father. His father had recently been treated successfully for paranoid schizophrenia. D.S. had visual and auditory hallucinations, was paranoid and very anxious. Differential diagnoses included alcoholic psychosis or schizophrenia. He was positive on the urine test and was treated as an alcoholic schizophrenic. He was given psychedelic therapy with 300 micrograms of LSD and later was started on niacin 3 grams daily. He was discharged April 26, 1960, and remained abstinent for six months. He was readmitted April 25, 1961. This time he received 5 ECT and the dose of niacin was doubled. After discharge, May 13, 1961, he remained well.

G.B., age 39, was alcoholic five years. There were no perceptual symptoms, but she was paranoid, tense, depressed, and suicidal. We had planned to treat her alcoholism with LSD. However, she was malvarian. We gave her LSD and started niacinamide the next day. She remained normal.

M.M., age 67, was a heavy drinker all his life, but had become much worse the previous three years. On closer examination it turned out he was not drinking more — his tolerance had gone down. He had a few mild perceptual symptoms and his thinking was disorganized. He was positive on the urine test. He was not given LSD; instead, he was started on niacin and recovered.

In contrast, alcoholics who were not schizophrenic or malvarian did not stop drinking when given vitamin B-3. Many other case histories on our study of malvaria, including depressions, personality problems, and retarded children, provided the same results.

The urine test is also helpful in determining prognosis. Patients who are positive for KP on discharge are not as well as those patients who are negative. Therefore, their prognosis after discharge is poorer, as shown in Table 18. Patients often became negative for KP after discharge and improved. Patients who remained positive did not recover in spite of the most intensive treatment.

I should add that we did not know KP caused a double deficiency of pyridoxine (vitamin B-6) and zinc. This was shown later by Dr Carl Pfeiffer. Thirty years ago we did not use vitamin B-6 and zinc in treatment. Had we given these

TABLE 18
Progress After Discharge for One Year Mean Follow-Up Period (One Month to Two Years)

	Positive	Negative
Number	23	20
Readmissions	31	10
Mean per patient	1.35	0.50
Last evaluation:		
Well	4	6
Much improved	7	7
Improved	5	4
Not Improved	7	3

patients large doses of pyridoxine and zinc as recommended by Dr Pfeiffer, we might have helped many more. We had found vitamin B-3 helpful and Dr Pfeiffer had found pyridoxine and zinc helpful. There is no clash of ideas here: Dr Pfeiffer also used vitamin B-3. Pyridoxine is essential in the conversion of tryptophan to vitamin B-3 in the body. Thus, a deficiency of vitamin B-6 would lead to a deficiency of vitamin B-3. Providing B-6 will overcome this deficiency, as will the provision of B-3. However, a deficiency of B-6 will have other consequences which will not be corrected by vitamin B-3. It appears that a deficiency of pyridoxine leads to the schizophrenic syndrome primarily because it causes a deficiency of vitamin B-3 and its coenzyme, NAD. Other signs of pyridoxine deficiency include changes in skin (white spots in fingernails, striae, acne, dry or oily skin), premenstrual problems, and more.

After re reading our early papers, I am more convinced than before that malvaria (now pyrroluria) is a valid schizophrenic syndrome, which is readily treated and responds well to orthomolecular treatment.

SCHIZOPHRENIC SYNDROMES

Cerebral Allergies

Drs Marshall Mandell and William Philpott introduced the concept of cerebral allergies into orthomolecular psychiatry in 1979. They demonstrated that allergic reactions could produce the schizophrenic syndrome, and that removing these reactions could cure them. This was difficult for psychiatrists to accept at first, for one of the "known" facts about schizophrenia was that it could not coexist with allergies. The concept of cerebral allergy points to the brain as the main target of the allergic reaction. It is easy to accept the concept when you have seen a schizophrenic become normal after a four or five day water fast, then relapse when the offending food or foods were reintroduced.

I have seen paranoid schizophrenics change in one hour from being calm, reasonable, cheerful people, to hostile, bitter, paranoid, over-excitable individuals, just from eating cheese. Once you witness this, you never forget it.

One of the first to describe this reaction was my old friend, Dr Walter Alvarez, head of gastroenterology, Mayo Clinic, Rochester, Minnesota. For many years after his retirement he wrote a very popular health column. He was hated by psychoanalysts because he very frequently lambasted their views in his column. His column was removed from the *New York Times* because senior *Times* editors were friendly with some analysts. Analysts always tried to suppress any criticism.

Around 1920, Dr Alvarez discovered why he felt "dumb" on Mondays. He realized it came from eating chicken on Sundays, the only day of the week he ate chicken. He stopped eating chicken and no longer felt dumb on Mondays. Chicken caused Dr Alvarez to suffer some confusion and some difficulty in thinking, which he described as feeling dumb. His paper created a problem; his colleagues were very disturbed about it because they knew no one could be allergic to foods. They exerted a lot of pressure to have him fired, until one day, one of the Mayo brothers came up to him and exclaimed, "Walter, best goddamn paper I have seen." After reading Alvarez' report, Dr Mayo was able to pinpoint one of his own allergies. The reaction of his colleagues 70 years ago is similar to the reaction of most physicians today, who can still not believe foods can cause schizophrenia.

In 1975 Dr Allan Cott successfully repeated the Russian fasting program for chronic schizophrenics. This inspired me to repeat this work. About 22 years ago I was asked to see a chronic schizophrenic woman. She was unable to come to my office because she was rigid, catatonic, so I went to see her at her home. She had been ill at least ten years and had not responded to treatment. I promptly delivered her to City Hospital, Saskatoon, by ambulance. Because she had been ill such a long time, I expected little response to vitamin therapy. She agreed to try a 30-day water fast. To my amazement she was well by the fifth day. I knew nothing about cerebral allergy and so continued her on the fast for another 25 days. She remained well and lost about 30 pounds. To my horror, a few days after she went off her fast her psychosis recurred.

During her fast she had felt so well that she begged me to allow her to do another long fast. I agreed to do so, but only after she had regained her weight. Once again, five days into her fast, she was well. By this time I was becoming more familiar with the cerebral allergy concept. I therefore terminated the fast and began to do individual food testing. She was allergic to all meats: as soon as she ate meat her major symptoms recurred. She then went on a vegetarian diet and remained well. Since then I have fasted at least 200 schizophrenic patients. They were all either failures from vitamin treatment or had only shown a partial response. More than 60 percent were well after the fast. Most of them were members of the cerebral allergy syndrome.

Cerebral allergies affect children as well, and can convert a young Dr Jekyll into a mean, miserable, obnoxious, hyperactive Mr. Hyde within minutes or hours. In adults, cerebral allergies may show up as schizophrenia; in children, learning and behavioral disorders, but they may also create other psychiatric syndromes such as mood swings from elation to depression.

Vitamin Deficiencies

Pellagra is the classical vitamin B-3 deficiency disease. It is caused by a monotonous diet deficient in vitamin B-3, deficient in l-tryptophan, and containing the wrong ratio of two other amino acids, leucine and isoleucine. Corn is the best example of a pellagra-producing food. It was very difficult to distinguish chronic pellagra from chronic schizophrenia until vitamin B-3 was identified as the anti-pellagra vitamin and became available. The vitamin would cure pellagrins. If they were thought to be schizophrenic and got well on vitamin B-3, they were reclassified as pellagra, and another schizophrenic syndrome was taken away from psychiatry. If the schizophrenia did not vanish, it remained a treatment failure — remained schizophrenia. We in psychiatry have always been left to deal with the failures. Early pellagrins got well on small doses of vitamin B-3, but chronic pellagrins needed 30 times as much, 600 mg per day, or more.

A deficiency of pyridoxine, vitamin B-6, can also cause schizophrenia: the body becomes unable convert enough l-tryptophan into NAD.

A pure deficiency of thiamine, B-1, will not cause schizophrenia. However, a combination of alcoholism and a B-1 deficiency is associated with a psychosis called Wernicke-Korsakoff. Usually one can distinguish this from schizophrenia, but sometimes they are indistinguishable. Several years ago a middle-aged woman with a long history of alcohol abuse was admitted, psychotic. Her family doctor diagnosed her as having Wernicke-Korsakoff disease. Her neurologist and psychiatrist concurred. She was declared untreatable and mentally incompetent. Her husband had heard about vitamin therapy and demanded I be consulted. She was referred to me and I, too, agreed she was suffering from Wernicke-Korsakoff. I started her on large doses of thiamine and niacin with no immediate response. Several weeks later I was in the hospital when I saw her almost catatonic and posturing, typical schizophrenic symptoms. I immediately reinvestigated her and discovered she had been treated for schizophrenia several years before, in a Vancouver hospital. I gave her three ECT and she became normal. I promptly initiated procedures to get her declared competent, and discharged her. She is still well, seven years later.

A deficiency of folic acid and vitamin B-12 will also cause psychosis, but this is infrequent and is more characteristic of the toxic psychoses.

Vitamin B-3 Dependency

There is no question that schizophrenics may require large doses of vitamin B-3. I am convinced they are cases of vitamin B-3 dependency — persons whose need for vitamin B-3 is so great, it cannot be met by diet alone. I am also convinced that if schizophrenics were started on vitamin B-3 before they became ill, during childhood, they would need much smaller doses, say less than 500 mg per day. If this is not provided, their needs will increase over time. Chronic patients certainly need larger doses than do acute patients. The situation is parallel to pellagra: early pellagrins respond to the usual vitamin (small) doses, but if they are sick for a long time, they will require much more. In the same way, dogs kept on a pellagra-producing diet for a short time get well on small doses of B-3. If kept on the deficient diet for six months or longer, they too will require larger doses: they will have become more dependent on the vitamin.

Mineral Deficiency

Zinc deficiency can produce a schizophrenic syndrome. It is probably a frequent complication of the pyridoxine deficiency syndrome, or pyrroluria. Dr Carl Pfeiffer described a girl in her mid-teens who recovered temporarily after a meal of oysters, which are very rich in zinc, and permanently on zinc salts. She had not responded to any previous treatment.

Mineral Toxicity

An excess of mercury, lead, copper, cadmium, or iron can cause psychotic reactions. Many years ago, before silver amalgams became common, only a few people suffered from mercury intoxication. Tradespeople using liquid mercury in making felt hats often became psychotic — mad hatters. Early in 1970 I saw two patients who became schizophrenic, both as a result of chronic exposure to mercury. This kind of exposure is rare, but exposure to mercury/silver dental amalgams (52 percent mercury when first installed) is ubiquitous; very few people have no fillings at all. In spite of violent protestations by the dental profession that these amalgams are safe, the evidence is very powerful that for many people they are unsafe. In Sweden, the government will pay the cost of removing mercury amalgams, and according to a program on the television show "60 Minutes," Germany plans to forbid their use. *The Journal of Orthomolecular Psychiatry* and *Journal of Orthomolecular Medicine* have carried original reports by Dr Hal Huggins and others about the danger of mercury from silver amalgams.

More attention has been given to lead toxicity which produces learning and behavioral disorders in children. However, I have not seen any adults suffering from lead poisoning.

Copper excess may also cause psychiatric problems, of which depression is the most common. It may also be associated with senility. I ran a series several years ago and found that in older patients blood copper levels went up from about 100 mcg/100mL to over 160 mcg/100mL. Patients with these high copper levels were most often depressed and complained of memory disturbances. Zinc levels did not go up or down with age.

The Hallucinogens

These are compounds such as mescaline, LSD, and even the amphetamines. The amphetamines tend to produce psychoses only after they have been used for a long time. LSD and mescaline cause acute short-lived reactions which are indistinguishable from schizophrenia. Vitamin B-3 will remove most of the LSD experience in a few minutes if given parenterally, and in an hour or so if taken orally.

TREATMENT

The cerebral allergy and vitamin dependency syndromes are the most common forms of schizophrenia. They should be investigated first. Eventually one may have to consider the possibility any one of the syndromes may be present and require treatment.

There are three phases of treatment, and all are utilized during the first interview. During the first phase the patient reports about matters on which he or she is an expert: symptoms, how they developed, and so on. The physician listens, records, and guides the narrative. For the patient it is really his story (history) or her story (herstory). During the second phase the doctor, using information only he or she knows, continues to question the patient, to elicit more pertinent information. During the third phase there is a general discussion between both physician and patient when diagnosis, possible causes, treatment and prognosis are examined in detail. At the end of the interview the patient should know what is wrong, how it came about, what to do, and what to expect. It is often best to have a close relative, friend, or confidante present since schizophrenic patients are often confused and preoccupied with their discomfort. I always record on my prescription pad the kind of diet, the supplements and their dosages, and the drugs and dosages I recommend for them.

Patients are seen again at regular intervals; the frequency depends upon the severity of the illness.

Most patients are already taking some medication at the time of the first interview. The medication was prescribed and monitored by their family doctor or by other psychiatrists they have seen. If the medication has been helpful and is not causing disturbing side effects, I maintain the same program. Vitamins usually require several months to kick in. If the drugs are stopped too soon, patients will relapse before they have a chance to note any beneficial effect from the vitamins.

There was, and still is, a common misconception that orthomolecular physicians are opposed to the use of medication and order patients to stop. I do not know where this strange idea came from, but I know it is held by many — patients have told me so. One physician who referred his patient to me warned the patient that it was my habit to stop all drugs immediately. Several years ago I received a letter from a Florida patient who wrote he had started to take vitamins for his schizophrenia. He also had stopped taking his tranquilizers. I wrote back that he must immediately get back onto his drugs. He showed my letter to his physician, who wrote to me expressing his surprise and thanking me.

Diet

Regardless of whether food allergies are suspected or not, I advise my patients to follow a sugar-free diet. This excludes any prepared foods to which sugars — table sugar, corn syrup, and so on — have been added. It therefore excludes most commercially prepared foods. It excludes almost all canned soups and other preparations, and most breakfast cereals. It does not exclude bread. The sugar added to dough is consumed by the yeast and is converted to alcohol, which is released during baking. The finished product should be sugar-free, unless it is a specialty sweet bread with extra sugar added. My patients in hospital are placed upon the same diet. Hospital food is generally typical institution food, not very nutritious. The sugar-free diet is more nutritious.

I exclude sugar because this is the easiest way I know to improve one's diet. The degree of improvement is a function of how bad it was before. If 50 percent of the calories are sugars, the 0 percent sugar diet will be a tremendous improvement. If only 5 percent of the calories come from added sugars, the improvement will be minimal. Fruit and dried fruit is allowed.

Patients find this diet rule easy to remember and fairly easy to follow. Children have more difficulty, and Christmas holidays are especially difficult. January is my relapse month. I then see patients who had been well suffering a resurgence of anxiety, depression, and other symptoms. September is the relapse month for children. Usually over the summer parents have less control over their children's food intake. The increase in sugar in their diet will in many cases return the child's pre-treatment behavior — usually hyperactivity.

Children cannot understand why something which tastes so good can be so harmful. They may accept the advice of the doctor and their parents, or they may refuse to go along. These children must realize by personal experience that sugar can be bad for them. One way of doing so is to reawaken a dormant reflex present in all mammals. If an animals eats a food and becomes very sick soon afterward, an association is made, and that animal will thereafter avoid that food. This "vomit" reflex is used to train animals not to hunt certain prey. To reduce the killing of sheep by coyotes, the wild animals have been given lamb meat containing enough lithium to make them nauseated. After eating the meat and becoming very ill, they will no longer hunt and kill lambs.

Children whose behavioral problems arise from their consumption of sugar are not made physically sick from their daily use of sweets. However, if they remain free of all sugar for at least 5 days and are then given a large amount of it, they may become physically ill with headache, abdominal pain, nausea, and sometimes vomiting. They then can draw the association between what they ate and how they felt afterward. If the child agrees, I place them on a weekly program. They must agree to avoid all sweets Monday through Friday. On Saturday they can eat as much as they like. I call this "Junk-Food Saturday." On Sunday they may still be ill, and by Monday they are back on the full program. After several such Saturdays, most children understand the connection and will thereafter avoid sweets. In my opinion, a high sugar intake increases the probability of developing allergies, not just to sugar but to other food as well.

Patients' food allergies often start very early in life, often when they have colic as infants. Colic is most often an allergy to cow's milk, or to mother's milk when the mother drinks large quantities of milk. Many women think drinking a lot of milk will help lactation and is good for them, but they may become allergic to milk. During infancy symptoms other than colic may develop. Babies start to have colds, runny nose, ear infections, and develop allergy shiners (dark swollen areas under their eyes), facial pallor from water retention, and a variety of learning and behavioral disorders. Later on, children may develop hay fever or asthma. In most cases adult allergies are not newly created: they can be traced back to childhood.

Usually, allergies develop to the staple foods. It is a

function of the amount consumed and the frequency. It is less usual to become allergic to foods eaten at intervals longer than 4 days. That is why a varied diet, which includes a large number of different foods, is much healthier than a monotonous diet.

If there is a history of allergy, one begins to look for the offending foods. Most physicians can go a long way in determining these foods using dietary clues and elimination diets. Favorite foods which are consumed often are apt to be the very ones to which the patient is allergic. Foods which cause definite adverse reactions are no problem and are easily avoided. However, dairy foods are an exception, and many patients have told me they can't stand milk but love cheese. In fact, before I discovered my own dairy allergy I had exactly the same view of milk and cheese. For as long as I can remember, I had used milk very sparingly — usually small amounts on my cereal, and I loved fermented cheese, but not cream or cottage cheese. I used to suffer three or four severe colds each year, each lasting up to a week. In 1966 I became interested in hypoglycemia, which called for a frequent-feeding, high protein diet, and I increased my intake of milk. One evening during a Chinese meal of won ton soup, I felt ill, my nose began to run, and I thought I was developing another cold. This one, however, lasted two years. I got no relief, no matter what I did. I then went onto a four day water fast, simply to experience what happened so I could discuss it more intelligently with my patients when I advised them to fast. I expected to have four unpleasant days, and this was true of the first three days, but to my amazement, on the fourth day I felt marvellous. My cold was gone and my nose was clear for the first time in two years. Now I could leave home for my office without pockets full of tissues. After taking some milk, my cold was back within a few minutes. Since then I have not knowingly taken any dairy products, but it has slipped into my food several times since. After each exposure I have another four day cold. Milk and its derivatives also produce phlegm and I get a sore throat.

Important clues to determining food allergies are these food likes and dislikes, and the quantity of these foods consumed. Another clue is how hungry one becomes after missing a meal. If the patient tells you he becomes weak and shaky after missing a meal, suspect a food allergy. I can go from several hours to several days without becoming unduly hungry. Another clue is the diurnal pattern of symptoms. If depression, fatigue, and nervousness come on only after certain meals, it may be due to the foods included in those meals. This is why food and associated symptom diaries can be very helpful. Another clue is the effect of sudden changes in diet. One of my patients returned from a holiday in Mexico. He told me that his symptoms, so troublesome at home, disappeared within a few days of his arrival in Mexico, and returned a few days after coming home. Canadians do not drink milk in Mexico. Neither did he. He had a milk allergy. On a milk-free diet at home, he recovered.

No matter what the clues are, the final test is clinical, the elimination diet. This may be a fast or any one of a number of diets, all designed to eliminate common animal products and staples. These diets are fully described in the book *Dr Mandell's 5-Day Allergy Relief System*. Eventually the offending food is eliminated, re-introduced, and eliminated, until the relationship is certain. Then the patient remains on the new allergy-free diet as well as being sugar-free.

Elimination diets are accurate, but they are tedious and time-consuming. It would be so much easier if we had laboratory tests which identified quickly those things to which we are allergic. Several tests are already available and their accuracy is improving. The more recent tests are very helpful. The tests include skin tests which are titered; i.e., they use various dilutions of the suspect allergens, or sublingual tests, or serological tests. The Elisa Test is very helpful. Patients may have many food allergies and these tests can be very helpful in working out what they are.

Vitamins in large doses may be very helpful for allergies. The most promising are niacin, niacinamide, and ascorbic acid. Niacin releases histamine from its storage cells in the body, and after it is dumped into the blood, it has a half-life of 90 minutes. The niacin flush is really a histamine flush. Prostaglandins also play a role. Niacin taken daily will gradually lower total histamine in the body, until there is not enough remaining in storage sites to cause flushing. Since histamine is released during allergic reactions and can cause toxic reactions, using niacin will decrease the intensity of these allergic reactions. This has not been tested in human subjects, but Dr E. Boyle found niacin protected guinea pigs from anaphylactic shock. Guinea pigs can be given one injection of a foreign protein with little effect, but if the same protein is injected a week later they will die from anaphylactic shock. However, after being treated with niacin, the second injection did not kill Dr Boyle's guinea pigs. All he could detect was that they wriggled their noses more. Niacin must be tested to see if it will protect people against the same type of shock.

I have seen how niacin reduces the intensity of reaction to insect bites. A friend of mine always got severe reactions to insect bites. A few days after taking niacin 3 grams per day, bites from the same insects caused only minor discomfort.

Finally, I am convinced that in large doses niacin will inhibit some of the allergic reactions to food. Some patients have needed large doses of niacin until they were placed on an elimination diet. After that, they could only tolerate much smaller doses. The food allergy increased their need for, and tolerance to, niacin. I have not noted niacinamide to be similarly useful, but other investigators have noted it has a beneficial effect.

Ascorbic acid destroys histamine. A massive discharge of histamine into the blood will therefore be less damaging when there is a lot of ascorbic acid circulating in the blood and present in the tissues of the body. Many years ago I was stung by a wasp. Immediately a hive developed, growing very quickly. I promptly took several grams of ascorbic acid by mouth and watched the hive. It continued to grow for a few more minutes, then stopped, and just as quickly diminished. Within one hour of being stung, I could see only a slight puncture site. The hive was entirely gone.

Dr Fred Klenner pioneered the use of large doses of ascorbic acid for many allergies. A review of its anti-allergy properties is available in Dr Stone's *The Healing Factor: Vitamin C against Disease* (1972) and Dr Pauling's *How To Live Longer and Feel Better* (1986). Dr Pauling's chapter on allergies reviews the medical literature. Evidence over the past 50 years shows the value of vitamin C in controlling allergic reactions. There is a close relationship between blood ascorbic acid and histamine levels. Guinea pigs on a scorbutic diet develop very high histamine levels in blood. This may be responsible for some of the symptoms of scurvy. In people, high levels of ascorbic acid in blood decrease histamine levels. The histamine level reaches a minimum with oral doses of vitamin C (over 250 mg per day). Stress also increases histamine levels. This is controlled by vitamin C. Ascorbic acid also protects guinea pigs against anaphylactic shock. A combination of niacin and ascorbate would be a very good anti-anaphylactic agent. As Dr Pauling recommends, "It would be wise for persons who might be exposed to agents that could cause anaphylaxis to ingest regular high doses of vitamin C."

Another compound, sodium chromoglycate, is helpful for occasional use. The dose is 100 mg, taken one hour before exposure to the food. If a patient wishes to eat the food and takes this compound, it will prevent most of the allergic reaction. Suppose you have a beef allergy but would like to go to a restaurant for a steak dinner. You would then use sodium chromoglycate to protect yourself against your usual reaction to beef. My patients use it in this way, but usually not on a steady basis.

Some patients have so many food allergies it is impossible to find an adequate diet for them. For these patients I use what I will call "non anti-depressant" doses of some of the modern tricyclic antidepressants, which are generally used at a dose range of 75 mg per day or more. At these doses it is common to have side effects — especially dry mouth. Clomipramine, also known as anafranil, is very helpful. I recommend 25 or 50 mg before bed. I have several patients who are now able to eat almost everything, whereas before they were unable to eat most foods. This is only surprising to those who are unaware that tricyclics are descended from antihistamines, and that they have good antihistaminic properties. This may be why they are so effective for patients who are clinically depressed; they are antihistamines which do not cause excessive drowsiness, as do most over-the-counter antihistamines.

A survey I did twenty-five years ago showed that about two-thirds of all people who were referred to me for depression had a history of allergies going back to childhood. A colleague in psychiatry who specialized in treating depression with drugs corroborated my findings on his own patients. I suspect these allergies are responsible for their depression. Patients who do not respond to tricyclics may not have allergies.

A combination of special diets tailored to a patient's own needs, the correct nutrients in optimum doses, and antidepressant drugs in a few cases will help most patients overcome their allergies. Several years ago, this approach helped a patient to recover. It required 75 mg per day of Anafranil before she stopped reacting to foods and her depression cleared. Two years later she stopped taking the antidepressant, and she remained normal for the following two years.

Suddenly she once more became allergic to so many foods that she could not maintain her caloric intake, and she began to lose weight from starvation. Her weight loss was so severe she was advised to start on a completely synthetic diet which provided all the nutrients, amino acids, glucose, fatty acids, vitamins, and minerals. These preparations are non-allergic and can be used to determine food allergies. Patients live on these preparations only for a week or more, and then add individual foods to test for reactivity. She was weak, very depressed, and anxious. She started back on Anafranil and within a month was well, no longer reacting to foods which a few weeks previous had made her violently ill.

Vitamin Supplements

The three main vitamins for treating schizophrenia are vitamin B-3, vitamin B-6, and vitamin C. Common starting doses are 3 grams daily of B-3, 3 grams daily of vitamin C, and 250 mg of vitamin B-6.

Vitamin B-1
(Thiamine)

The amount of thiamine present in B-complex preparations is adequate for most people. The B-complex 50s contain 50 mg per tablet of thiamine, niacinamide, pyridoxine, and pantothenic acid. The main indication for larger doses of B-1 is alcoholism. Patients with Wernicke-Korsakoff syndrome need a lot more. It was also used by Dr Fred Klenner in the treatment of multiple sclerosis. I believe that people who consume large amounts of sugars should also take extra thiamine.

Vitamin B-3
(Niacin and Niacinamide)

Both forms of vitamin B-3 are effective for treating the schizophrenias, but there are differences. Niacin is a peripheral vasodilator which causes flushing of the skin, beginning in the face. The first time niacin is taken, the reaction is the most intense. In time, most people get used to it and stop flushing, unless they stop using it for a few days. This flush is irritating to many people, and does limit the use of niacin.

I usually start people out on niacinamide, which does not cause any flushing. If it seems to be less effective after an adequate trial period, I will then advise that niacin be used instead. Niacin can be taken in larger doses before nausea develops. There is a nauseant dose for both forms of B-3. Few people can tolerate more than 6 grams of niacinamide per day, but many can take doses of niacin up to 12 grams and more, daily.

Niacin is better for many people because it may be therapeutic more quickly, and because higher doses can be given with few or no side effects. Occasionally niacin is much more effective. A few months ago I took a patient off niacinamide who had been taking it for three months with little response. Four days after starting niacin she was normal, according to her father, and this was confirmed by her friends.

I prefer to use niacin and niacinamide as follows:

ᕙ 1. For children, niacinamide, unless they dislike the bitter taste or have too low a nauseant threshold. Children often will not complain of nausea but will lose their appetite without complaining about it. They are then given niacin instead. They often prefer niacin's sour taste, and can easily tolerate adult doses.

ᕙ 2. For patients who do not want to be seen flushing for cosmetic reasons, I start with niacinamide. I will switch to niacin if the response is too slow or if there are side effects such as nausea.

ᕙ 3. For aging patients I prefer to start with niacin. It works more efficiently, improves circulation, and normalizes cholesterol levels.

❧ 4. When the nauseant dose is too small for either form of vitamin B-3, I use them in combination; i.e., if the nauseant dose is 2 grams per day for each, I will use 1.5 grams of niacin with 1.5 grams of niacinamide to give a total vitamin B-3 dose of 3 grams per day.

The niacin flush may be a problem for patients, but if patients are prepared for it and if their physicians are knowledgeable, it can be minimized, and very seldom needs to be discontinued. It is absolutely essential patients are told what to expect. If they are caught unaware, they may panic, and will in most cases not want to take any more. There have been many examples of patients calling hospital emergency departments for help. A man in Detroit, at the height of the flush, called a poison control center and was told he had taken a toxic dose. But during the ambulance ride to hospital he recovered. The intensity of the niacin flush generally depends upon the degree of need, and from my experience, patients who need niacin most have the least initial flush reaction.

The reaction (vasodilation) can be minimized by some of the following techniques:

❧ 1. By taking the niacin right after a meal with a cold drink. Niacin is absorbed quickly, especially when taken with a hot liquid. Maximum flush would be obtained by drinking a hot solution of niacin.

❧ 2. By continued, regular doses of niacin. Niacin itself is the best anti-flush preparation. If it is not taken for a few days, the flush mechanism is reactivated. However, many people do not ever become accustomed to the flush, and they will have to use niacinamide or a timed-release preparation, or one of the niacin esters such as inositol niacinate. The esters are the best non-flushing forms of niacin.

TABLE 19
Vitamin B-3 Dose Range Recommended

Disease	Daily Range (Usually in three doses daily for higher doses)
Anti-pellagra (minimal good health)	20 to 30 mg
Anti-pellagra for chronic pellagrins	500–1000 mg
Anti-subclinical pellagra (for optimal good health)	100–1000 mg
Anti-psychotic, schizophrenia, deliria, LSD psychosis	1–12 grams
To normalize cholesterol levels	1.5–9 grams
Anti-arthritic	0.5–6 grams
Children with learning and behavioral disorders	1–3 grams
Anti-cancer	100–3000 mg
Anti-aging	1500–6000 mg
Miscellaneous	100–3000 mg

3. By the use of antihistamines. These compounds decrease the intensity of the flush and may even eliminate it. It is most likely that it is the release of histamine in the body which is responsible for causing the flush.

4. Aspirin begun a few days in advance of starting on niacin also decreases the intensity of the flush. Other prostaglandin antagonists have similar properties. The usual dose of aspirin is one or two 325 mg tablets per day, starting two days before going onto niacin.

༳ 5. By the way the flush is described to the patient. A complete description of the flushing sequence, followed by an outline of reasons why it is being recommended, will be very helpful. Physicians who do not like niacin seldom find their patients can tolerate it, while physicians who find it very useful have little problem. A few patients enjoy the flush and will go off it for a few days in order to reactivate it. This occurs with arthritics more frequently than with other conditions.

I generally start patients on 3 grams of B-3 per day, using 500 mg tablets. Thereafter the dose is evaluated at each follow-up interview. If the patient makes significant progress, the dose remains the same. If there are side effects, it is decreased. If there is too little progress, I will increase the dose to 6 grams. In each case, the maximum dose is reached when nausea develops. If there is nausea, the B-3 is reduced or discontinued, because if it is continued, it will lead to vomiting. One day we will have a number of niacinate compounds which will be effective in lower doses, with fewer side effects. See Table 19 for recommended dosages.

Maintenance doses may be a lot lower than initial therapeutic doses. Many patients have remained well on 1 gram per day. Patients should learn as much as they can about their own illness. After patients have been well long enough, they may consider stopping the vitamin, but at the first indication the illness may be returning, should resume treatment.

Vitamin B-6
(Pyridoxine)

The main indication for vitamin B-6 is pyrroluria, shown by Dr Carl Pfeiffer to be a double deficiency of pyridoxine and zinc. It can be diagnosed using clinical criteria. The dose ranges up to 2 grams daily, but I have seldom needed to go higher than 750 mg daily. It is available in 250 mg tablets. Pyridoxine is also valuable for the treatment of infantile autism, as shown by more than one dozen double-blind controlled experiments. It works best when taken in combination with zinc, and for some children magnesium is needed as well, because pyridoxine alone may increase irritability.

Vitamin C
(*Ascorbic Acid*)

I usually give 3 grams daily of vitamin C but may increase the dose to bowel tolerance levels. This is the dose which causes gas and loose bowels. The bowel tolerance level varies enormously from person to person, and even for the same person over time. Because it loosens bowel movements, it is valuable for people who suffer from constipation. The dose is increased until the patient is content with their bowel frequency — twice per day is optimal. I also consider vitamin C a very important anti-stress nutrient.

The optimum dose of ascorbic acid depends upon the nature of the illness — severe diseases require much higher doses. For the treatment of cancer, the minimum dose is 12 grams per day. Dr Fred Klenner used doses up to 100 grams per day. In many cases it is best given intravenously as mineral ascorbates.

I have rarely given schizophrenic patients huge doses, say 40 grams per day or more. I think it should be done; this was a major oversight. The first time I gave a patient more than 3 grams daily occurred in 1952. I had ample supplies of pure ascorbic acid and was running clinical tests using different doses. A middle-aged woman was admitted, psychotic. Her psychiatrist diagnosed her as being schizophrenic and arranged to start ECT the following Monday. For reasons I don't remember now, I wanted to try out ascorbic acid. She had become psychotic after unsuccessful treatment for breast cancer. After surgery the lesion would not heal and was ulcerated. I had no clinical interest in her cancer, only in her mental state. I had hoped to give her 3 grams per day for a couple of weeks at least. Her psychiatrist agreed I could give her vitamin C, but would not withhold the ECT. I therefore had only 48 hours. I was certain 3 grams could do little in two days and so decided to give her 1 gram every hour.

By Monday morning she had received 45 grams over a two day period. I was pleased that she showed no side effects — and was very surprised because she was no longer psychotic. Her doctor did not give her ECT and discharged her from hospital one week later. We also noted that the lesion had become less inflamed and had started to heal. She was not given any follow-up vitamin after discharge. She died six months later from her cancer, but remained mentally normal. At that time it did not occur to me to follow up the remarkable finding that her breast lesion had started to heal.

After we became preoccupied with our double-blind controlled experiments, I made a few sporadic studies with vitamin C, using it as an anti-tension compound. There were two striking responses. The first was a young, chronic schizophrenic woman who had responded only partially to ECT, vitamin B-3, and tranquilizers. She became extremely tense and agitated. The only way she could relieve her tension was to pace the corridor of the hospital, hour after hour. She wore out the heels of her shoes and began to damage her feet. One day I started her on vitamin C, 10 grams daily. Within a few days her anxiety and tension had subsided. She became normal and is still well today, about thirty years later.

My second patient came from Vancouver to Saskatoon, where I treated her with vitamin B-3 and ECT. She was a lot better and returned to her home in Vancouver. A few years later she relapsed and returned to Saskatoon for a repeat series of ECT. Shortly after I moved to Victoria in 1976, she again consulted me with a recurrence of her psychosis. One of her most distressing symptoms was a sensation that half her brain was dead. She demanded another series of ECT, stating that of all the treatments she had ever had, it was the only thing that had given her any relief. I gave her another series of ECT. A few months later she demanded another series. By now I was determined I would not give her any more if I could help it. I told her I would not give her any more and she immediately became even more depressed. Then I advised her to take ascorbic acid 10 grams per day. She reluctantly agreed to do so, convinced only ECT would help. One month later she was well; that dreadful sensation of her brain being half dead was gone. She has not been back since, and has remained well.

Mineral Supplements

I will discuss the nutrient supplements unique to orthomolecular treatment. Other minerals are well known to physicians and include iodine for hypothyroid problems, iron for iron deficiency anemia, calcium for osteoporosis, pregnancy and lactation, potassium and sodium.

Zinc

A deficiency of zinc is more common than is generally recognized. Zinc is leached from water-washed soils and is removed when grains are milled. One of the richest sources of zinc is oysters, not generally a staple food. I routinely use zinc in association with pyridoxine for schizophrenia. I use larger doses for elderly patients who have problems with their sense of smell or taste. A zinc deficiency removes normal sensations of taste and foods become flat or bitter, or taste foul. This can be life-threatening, as patients lose all appetite for food and may starve. I am convinced many elderly people suffer from zinc deficiency. I also use zinc for men developing prostate enlargement, and in many cases this will halt the enlargement process.

Zinc is also useful in reducing elevated copper levels. There is evidence it can be used successfully in treating Wilson's disease. Cuprimine, a copper chelator, was formerly used; zinc is safer.

Various zinc salts are available, including gluconate, citrate, and sulfate. I use between 25 and 100 mg per day. A few people may require a liquid form — a solution of zinc sulfate, which is easily made up by pharmacists. I recommend a solution of 10 percent zinc sulfate with .5 percent manganese chloride, as developed by Dr Carl Pfeiffer.

A zinc sulfate solution can be useful in measuring a deficiency of zinc. A person with normal zinc levels, when given a teaspoonful of this solution, will detect a sharp bitter taste almost immediately. Zinc deficient individuals may never taste it. The rapidity of the response and the intensity of the bitter taste are good measures of zinc deficiency. One can also use blood and hair assays.

Manganese

I use this mineral to prevent and treat tardive dyskinesia. Dr Richard Kunin discovered in 1976 that tardive dyskinesia is caused by a deficiency of manganese. Tardive dyskinesia is caused by tranquilizers and may affect up to 40 percent of schizophrenic patients. It was considered untreatable. However, early cases do recover if the tranquilizer is removed, but often it is better for the patient to remain on the tranquilizer. These complex molecules bind manganese and cause the deficiency. The addition of manganese will prevent tardive dyskinesia from developing. I have seen patients with severe tardive dyskinesia lose their tremor and other symptoms within a few days of starting manganese. Orthomolecular psychiatrists never produce new cases of tardive dyskinesia, the only ones they see are patients who come to them all ready suffering from it. I consider tardive dyskinesia an iatrogenic (doctor-caused) disease. There is no longer any excuse for patients and their families to have to suffer this complication of tranquilizer medication.

Magnesium

Magnesium and calcium should be given together. Orthomolecular physicians use a ratio of calcium to magnesium of 2 to 1 or 1 to 1. Magnesium tends to relax muscles. It is also needed by a few hyperactive children who are given pyridoxine. Generally calcium/magnesium supplements are needed for patients with special needs, such as during pregnancy or lactation. A diet which contains moderate amounts of protein and is free of additives will usually contain enough calcium and magnesium. There is probably a weak association between osteoporosis and calcium and magnesium levels.

Amino Acid Supplements

Two amino acids are associated with orthomolecular psychiatric practice: l-tryptophan and l-tyrosine. Some of the other amino acids have been used experimentally, but have not been generally accepted.

L-tryptophan is used for treatment of insomnia, as a natural sedative, and, more recently, as a treatment for bipolar mood disorders (manic-depressive psychosis). Taken on an empty stomach or with carbohydrate, it crosses the blood/brain barrier where some of it is converted to serotonin. This induces sleep in about 50 percent of patients, without any morning hangover. I first became aware of its relaxant properties in 1956, when I took a 5 gram dose to study its effect. I developed the same sensation I normally had after a 1 ounce drink of whiskey.

In the past few years I have used l-tryptophan in doses of 2 grams three times per day to treat manic-depressives who could not tolerate lithium. It has worked very well, with no side effects. Some of the l-tryptophan made in Japan and available in the U.S. contained a toxic contaminant which caused some deaths. The FDA removed all l-tryptophan from health food stores, and at this time, even though it is known what went wrong, it has not been released. Authorities tend to deal more harshly with nutrients than they do with drugs. In Canada, where l-tryptophan is available by prescription under the trade name Tryptan, it was not removed from drug stores, and no cases of Tryptan toxicity have been reported in Canada.

L-tryptophan should be very effective for schizophrenic patients who also have mood swings. Psychiatrists tend to diagnose these patients manic-depressive, overemphasizing the mood symptoms and ignoring symptoms of perceptual and thought disorder. This, then, justifies their use of lithium, which is recognized as a valuable treatment for manic-depressive disorders. This supposition is not logically supported, since one cannot use response to a drug as a measure of diagnosis. Schizophrenia with mood disorders can respond to lithium, which will help control mood.

I have observed that on orthomolecular treatment mood disorder generally disappears after several years. If only lithium is used, patients may need to take it forever. In combination with vitamin B-3, l-tryptophan may be even more effective as a source of serotonin, for by the chemical law of mass action, having a lot of vitamin B-3 in the body will force more l-tryptophan into serotonin.

L-tyrosine is used for treating depression. Tyrosine is a sympathomimetic amine, as are noradrenalin and adrenalin. They are activators. One of the explanations for the antidepressant properties of modern drugs is that they increase the effect of noradrenalin in the nervous system. L-tyrosine is given in the early part of the day and l-tryptophan toward the latter part of the day. This treatment is described by Dr Priscilla Slagle in her book, *The Way Up From Down*. I have a patient on this program now, and she has been stable for the past several months. She is also on an elimination diet, and on vitamin and mineral supplements.

Essential Fatty Acids (EFA)

There are two classes of essential fatty acids, Omega-3 EFA and Omega-6 EFA. The Omega-3 series are more unsaturated, i.e., have more double bonds or less hydrogen. They are described well in the work of Dr Donald Rudin and in Dr David Horrobin's book *Omega 6 Essential Fatty Acids*.

Both classes of EFA are essential for good health. Modern foods have been refined and these EFA have been removed. Diets should be improved by avoiding foods which are hydrogenated or deprived of their natural EFA. The best sources for the Omega-3 series are northern (cold climate) foods, fish, etc., and the best supplement is flaxseed (linseed) oil. The oil is very rich in Omega-3 EFA. I use one to four tablespoons daily, or use freshly ground flaxseed in cereal. The Omega-6 group are not as likely to be deficient, but there may be a problem in converting linolenic acid to gamma linolenic acid. Evening primrose oil is very helpful. There is a very large literature describing the clinical use of evening primrose oil.

Electroconvulsive Therapy (ECT)

It is almost impossible to discuss ECT in a rational way anymore. There is a loud, hostile, anti-ECT group, consisting of ex-ECT patients and a very small number of physicians, who are violently opposed to its use. Their reasoning is entirely out of context, and much of their argument is driven by the word "shock," not by the treatment itself. ECT, like any medical or surgical procedure, must be used carefully. When it is so used, it is a very effective treatment for a very small proportion of patients with severe depression and/or schizophrenia.

Before the full spectrum of orthomolecular treatment was available to me, I had to use ECT much more frequently, but over the past few years fewer than 1 percent of my patients have required it. Almost all of these patients have recovered, are grateful they are well, and would take ECT again if they relapsed back to their previous sick state.

For some time after a series of ECT there is a memory problem. This difficulty is almost completely removed if niacin is given with the ECT. I recall the first time I made this observation. In 1951 a woman brought her husband in to hospital because for the months since his last ECT, he could not remember anything and was confused. I had no treatment and would normally have counselled her to be patient and wait for this effect to leave. I was then just becoming very interested in niacin and decided I could not harm him with this safe vitamin. He began to take 3 grams per day. One month later, both husband and wife were happy: he was normal, and his wife was relieved and grateful. I have not given any ECT over the past thirty-five years unless patients are also receiving niacin.

Critics have complained about the use of ECT by orthomolecular physicians because they declare ECT is not orthomolecular. Of course, since no one knows why ECT is effective, they may be wrong. It certainly does correct some biochemical abnormality because patients are improved or cured. All we need to assume is that the presence of symptoms is a measure of metabolic abnormality.

Drugs

There are three main classes of drugs: (a) tranquilizers, (b) anti-anxiety drugs, and (c) antidepressants. The distinction between these drugs classes is not sharp, and any one drug of a certain class can affect all three areas.

Tranquilizers

Tranquilizers, because they are toxic, differ markedly from compounds normally present in the body, but in sub toxic (therapeutic) doses, they may be very valuable. Still, the side effects and toxicity of the tranquilizers make it impossible for patients to become normal while taking them. I call this the "tranquilizer dilemma."

The first tranquilizer, chlorpromazine (thorazine in the U.S.), was introduced in 1951. It is a direct descendant of the phenothiazine antihistamines such as benadryl. Since that time, a large number of tranquilizers have been introduced, each one with slightly different properties and with differences in side effects and dosages required. Basically, their main function is to diminish what I have called "hot" symptoms. All the symptoms of schizophrenia can be classed as "hot" or "cool." Hot symptoms cause major changes in behavior which characterize the schizophrenic syndrome; for example, hallucinations are hot, while illusions are cool. That is because hallucinations will most often lead to unusual behavior. Illusions are subtle and less often cause behavior which can be recognized as psychotic. In the area of thinking, delusions are hot. Thought blocking, memory problems, and difficulty with concentration are cool. Cool symptoms will influence behavior, but not to the same degree as delusions.

Recently, in my office, a paranoid patient began to tell me about his very bizarre ideas; for example, that Hitler had captured the souls of five million people and was working with these now. He was full of other bizarre ideas. I told him I was really not very interested in these ideas. He suddenly became very loud, began to shout at the top of his voice, and eventually smashed his fist down on my desk. The desk rebounded from the floor. Then he settled down. A few days later, under the influence of tranquilizers, he was quiet and no longer preoccupied with his paranoid delusions. The tranquilizers had cooled down his hot symptoms. In mood, hot symptoms are agitation and restlessness; mood which is flat or depressed is cool. Tranquilizers tend to cool these hot symptoms down, but they have no effect on cool symptoms, and may even make them worse.

The continued presence of cool symptoms prevents the patient from becoming well. We should have realized this thirty-five years ago because we knew then that tranquilizers made schizophrenics better and made normal people sick. One of the first animal tests for tranquilizer activity was the production of catatonia in animals.

Tranquilizers given to a patient soon cool down the hot symptoms, and the patient feels improved and appears to be better. As the hot symptoms recede into the background, the remaining cool symptoms become predominant. In other words, as the patient becomes better he begins to respond to the tranquilizers as if he were normal, i.e., by being made sick. On the continuum between disease and good health, tranquilizers move the patient closer and closer to being well. But it then becomes ever more difficult to reach normality, as the patient reacts to the tranquilizer more and more as would any other normal person, by being impaired by the drug. The best modern example of normal people being made sick by tranquilizers were the Russian dissidents, committed to mental hospitals and forced to take drugs.

Psychiatrists cope with the tranquilizer induced cool symptoms by decreasing the dose or discontinuing the drug. This would be good, except that the basic schizophrenic process is still burning actively, and will again become hot if the drug is removed, or the dose lowered too far. Patients cope with the problem of cool symptoms by refusing to take medication. They forget what it was like with their hot symptoms, and find the cool symptoms plus the tranquilizer side effects intolerable. Psychiatrists get around this by using injections of long-acting drugs. One injection will work for two to four weeks. The mental hospital revolving-door phenomenon is due to the reduction of hot symptoms by drugs which leads to discharge, followed by the re-emergence of hot symptoms when patients stop the drugs, which in turn forces them back into hospital.

Tranquilizers have the following physical and psychiatric side effects. Physical effects include tremor, loss of coordination, weakness, lethargy, decrease in concentration, difficulty with memory, and, in several cases, tardive dyskinesia and impotence. Psychiatric effects include loss of motivation, disinterest, loss of creativity. The end result is a patient who is unable to work, on welfare, and probably spends too much time watching TV. This syndrome makes up the tranquilizer psychosis, which is almost as disabling as the original psychosis.

In short, schizophrenic patients oscillate between schizophrenia and the tranquilizer psychosis, with the drugs driving them one way and the pressure of the disease driving them back if the drug is removed. The patient must choose between one of two psychoses, both unpleasant.

With orthomolecular psychiatry, this dilemma does not exist. As the patient's psychosis recedes, nutrients take over and eventually the patient can remain well while continuing on the nutrients. Tranquilizers are then either not needed, or are needed in such low dosages there are no side effects.

In orthomolecular therapy, the tranquilizers are used in the usual way. One starts out with an effective dose, maintaining that dose until the nutrition and supplements begin to show an effect. Then the drugs are very slowly and carefully reduced. In combination with vitamin B-3, tranquilizers are more effective, meaning that lower doses of drugs are as effective as the higher doses required when vitamin B-3 is not used. This decreases the intensity of side effects and allows the patient to be more comfortable and, even more important, to be more functional. The use of vitamin B-3 solves the tranquilizer dilemma.

Just why vitamin B-3 potentiates the effect of tranquilizers is not known. Perhaps it does not; on the contrary, it may be that tranquilizers potentiate the effect of vitamin B-3 so that less tranquilizer is needed. Many years ago investigators found that tranquilizers increase the interval during which high levels of NAD are maintained in red blood cells. After niacin or niacinamide is given, it is converted into its coenzyme, nicotinic acid dinucleotide (NAD). The amount of NAD in the red blood cells increases and, after a few minutes, starts to decrease. If vitamin B-3 is given at the same time, the levels of NSD stay elevated much longer. Since NAD is the active compound and is involved in most of the reactions in the body, elevated levels are therapeutic. The elevation in red blood cells suggests NAD is elevated in all cells, but this has not been tested. I remain amazed that this remarkable finding has been totally ignored for several decades.

Over the past thirty-five years I have not seen many patients recover on tranquilizers alone, although a proportion of patients will become much better and thereafter can get along without a tranquilizer. This is the group who naturally tend to get well, the natural (untreated) recovery rate being around 15 to 25 percent. They would have gotten well anyway, and this is accelerated by the drug. But if patients must remain on tranquilizers, they will not be well, nor will they be able to carry on any normal activity apart from the simplest, routine jobs.

The ideal treatment is to follow the orthomolecular approach. If the symptoms are too hot, tranquilizers are added. This combination allows one to take advantage of the rapidity of the response to tranquilizers, with the curative properties of the nutrients. Some day it will be malpractice not to use this approach, for schizophrenia is certainly not due to a deficiency of tranquilizers, but most syndromes are caused by a deficiency and/or dependency of natural molecules normally present in the body.

Antidepressants

These chemicals do not create anything equivalent to the tranquilizer psychosis. They are used as needed and are perfectly compatible with the orthomolecular approach. Their use in treating allergies has all ready been described.

I also use antidepressants in a way I have not seen described by other physicians. About twenty years ago it occurred to me that I had never seen a paranoid patient who was happy. Paranoid patients are depressed, tense, irritable, suspicious, and often unfriendly. I reasoned that if this was a true phenomenon, then one could remove paranoid symptoms by using antidepressants to remove their depression. I also realized that paranoid ideas recur over and over, and in this way are very similar to obsessive-compulsive symptoms. Anafranil is one of the best anti obsessive-compulsive antidepressants.

I therefore gave anafranil to one of my chronic paranoid schizophrenic patients. He had been in treatment for many years and was improved, but nothing I had tried would remove his paranoid ideas. He was so suspicious that children playing half a block away and making the usual noise indicated to him they were doing it to injure him. I started him on anafranil, 75 mg per day. There was no change for three months, then his paranoid ideas began to subside. Within two years they were almost gone and had taken a more benign course. He has been on Anafranil over sixteen years and is still much better. There has been no need to increase the dose. Since that time I have routinely given anafranil to my paranoid patients. In most cases it is very helpful. I am convinced it is impossible to be both paranoid and cheerful simultaneously.

Anti-Anxiety Drugs

In this class of drugs I include compounds like the diazepines. They are helpful in the short run, but have to be monitored as it is relatively easy to become dependent on them.

Psychiatric Treatment

So far I have described what I call the "medical" treatment of disease using diet, supplements, and drugs. This does not mean I ignore the doctor-patient relationship, which I consider the "psychiatric" part of treatment. Most patients early in their illness, who have not been deteriorated by the disease, require minimal psychiatric treatment. The psychiatric portion of their treatment includes diagnosing, telling the patient the diagnosis, and describing what the illness is — a biochemical malfunction or disease. Then, treatment is outlined in detail and prognosis is discussed. All the patient's questions are answered. In fact, questions are encouraged. Patients are also encouraged to read about schizophrenia, using material available from the Canadian Schizophrenia Foundation. After that, treatment is followed, patients are supported, and provision is made to deal with problems which arise during treatment.

Chronic patients will require much more psychiatric treatment, and also other therapy from a variety of specialists. They will need help from social workers, psychologists, nurses, counselors, etc. They may require special education or re-education, and many require special training in life skills, for jobs, or rehabilitation. Ideally, every resource will be used to restore normality to patients who have been severely damaged by the disease. Special homes, such as group homes, are often required. However, none of these professionals will get anywhere until orthomolecular treatment is introduced, and it may take several years before patients recover enough to really benefit from the other types of care. Not every patient can be recovered, but certainly no acute patient should be allowed to become chronic. Tranquilizers do not prevent chronicity; orthomolecular therapy does.

Not only is current orthomolecular treatment superior to traditional drug and psychoanalytical therapy, but also

TABLE 20

Group	Duration of Treatment	Well and Much Improved
A. Sick one year, or in second or third relapse.	Up to 1 year	90%
B. Sick 2–5 years.	Up to 5 years	75%
C. Sick over 5 years, but out of mental hospital.	5 or more years	50%
D. Sick over 5 years and in mental hospital.	5 or more years	25%

to our original vitamin B-3 therapy. I now expect the results shown in Table 20 from orthomolecular therapy.

VITAMIN B-3 AND MENTALLY DISTURBED CHILDREN

In 1954 I began a double-blind experiment with children comparing niacin and placebo. Of course, this was not truly double-blind since it is impossible to blind niacin, but does compare with the Canadian Mental Health Association-supported Montreal studies by Professor H. Lehmann. Nineteen students from a school for retarded children were selected. They were given placebo or niacin 1 gram per 50 pounds body weight, for three months. At the end of the study, parents and teachers reported any improvement. Out of 11 children on placebo, 3 were judged to be better, but out of 8 children on niacin, 7 were so judged. This difference was significant at the 5 percent level. I had not reported the results of my study, unlike the authors of the Montreal study, because it was not truly double-blind.

Later, in Saskatoon, I conducted a study with niacinamide on 24 children selected from a local school for retarded children. All were tested for kryptopyrrole, the mauve factor. Parents were not told the results of the urine test. The children were given niacinamide 1 gram per 50 pounds body weight for one year. I assumed that if the children improved, parents would continue to ask for their free supply of the vitamin. At the end of the year, out of the 16 who did not have kryptopyrrole, 5 were still on the vitamin, but from the kryptopyrrole-positive group all were still using the vitamin. These parents were optimistic and reported that their children were quieter, less aggressive, and learning better. Chi Square for this difference was 7.5; i.e., the probability that this was due to chance was less than 1 percent.

Since then I have given vitamin B-3, either alone or in combination with other nutrients, to over 1500 children under age 14, and the results have remained much superior to any other treatment. The treatment today is more sophisticated and comprehensive, and the results are even better. In fact, I rarely see failures on this treatment, and when they do occur, it is usually because these children and their families were unable to stay on the program long enough.

I had forgotten how long ago it was when I first started to use vitamin B-3 for children. In 1986 I rediscovered my first child, M.G., whom I first saw in June 1951 at a children's clinic. She was five years old at the time and was still not speaking well. She sat up at four months and walked by eleven months. There had been no birth injury or childhood diseases to account for this delay, and she had been breast fed. M.G. was a quiet, passive baby. She used a few words at age 3 and by age 4 years knew about 20 words, mostly Spanish, which she learned from a Spanish maid. When I saw her, she knew about 200 words. She would speak when she was interested, but if she was asked to repeat a word would block or mumble. Yet, according to an IQ test, she was normal.

In the fall of 1951, in grade one, she learned to read and was promoted to grade two, later to grade three. By July 1954 she had deteriorated. She was hyperactive and a very restless sleeper. She spoke in bursts, laughed too loudly and excessively. She tried to participate in groups, but when she was rejected, she withdrew, remaining at the edge of the group talking to her doll. Her thinking was concrete and her arithmetic was very poor. She spent a lot of time talking out loud to herself, repeating real events chiefly about enemies. I concluded she was schizophrenic and started her on niacin 1 gram per 50 pounds of body weight.

By November 1954 she was more curious, asked more questions, and occasionally joked when playing with her parents. (I have observed over the years that on vitamin B-3 often the first indication of improvement is the development of a sense of humor and smiling appropriately.) She was calmer and played better with children. Because her progress was so slow, she was sent to a special school in June 1955.

By fall 1957, because her progress was still slow, niacin was withheld for three months without informing her teachers; only the school director and her parents were aware of this. By the end of this trial period she had regressed. She had lost her spontaneity and exuberance. In February 1958 she was started back on niacin, again without her teachers' knowledge, and by April that year the consensus was that she was much better again. She remained on the vitamin.

In December 1962 the school reported, "In the classroom she is normally very quiet and attentive. However, she at times seems preoccupied and pressure is required to regain her attention. She is somewhat self-conscious and does not always react positively to correction. She completes all assignments, but does not initiate work independently. She participates eagerly in all phases of the recreational program. She requires leadership in organized activities but she is always very cooperative and exhibits a sense of fair play. She seems to particularly enjoy the square dance classes in which she has done very well."

She had spent this summer with her family. She got on well with them and was reluctant to go back to school in the fall. She had several arguments with her sister, $1^1/2$ years her junior (age $14^1/2$). These were normal teen arguments and she had held her own. According to her family, she related well to other teenagers. She loved to talk and would carry on long conversations with them about her school and popular music. She had a very good memory. With strangers her behavior was appropriate, but at sixteen her behavior was more that of a normal fourteen-year-old. Her mother wrote, "She is well developed, pretty with a nice figure, weighing 125 pounds at 5 feet 3 inches tall. Her skin is clear and glowing, and she has brown wavy hair. She falls asleep quite promptly and does not waken abnormally early as she used to." It is clear she was a little behind in her social development, but was within the normal range of teenage behavior.

This patient represents the best possible treatment of that day. It included vitamin B-3 to correct her metabolic abnormality, combined with special education in a residential school, with excellent understanding and support from her family. Had any one of these components been neglected, she would not have had this happy outcome.

Today she would have been placed on a special diet supplemented by other nutrients. I am convinced her progress would have been faster and that she would not have needed to attend that special school. Fewer than five percent of all the schizophrenic children I have treated need to have special instruction, and none have had to go to residential schools for children with learning or behavioral disorders.

Two other children were started on treatment in 1060. One is now a research physician, the other is a teacher, happily married with her own family. Since they received vitamin B-3 only, their histories are instructive.

In 1960 a physician called me from the United States, very depressed and weeping. His son, age thirteen, had been in a university hospital psychiatric ward for several months. This father had been advised by the professor of psychiatry that there was no treatment for his son, that he would never recover, and that it would be best for the family to commit him to a mental hospital and forget him as soon as possible.

However, this man could not accept this advice. He began to search in the medical library and ran across our first major report from 1957. He was able to locate Humphry Osmond, who advised him to call me at University Hospital in Saskatoon. During my conversation with him, I discussed with him what he might do, telling him that if he were my son, I would put him on niacin 3 grams per day. I suggested he use 500 mg tablets to avoid the toxic effects of the fillers present in the 100 mg tablets. He located a small vitamin company in Oregon that agreed to make up 500 mg tablets for him. They were the first company to provide 500 mg tablets of niacin for sale.

As soon as this doctor got the supply of niacin, he took a bottle of them to the hospital and requested his son be started on it. The professor of psychiatry became very hostile, stating that the had already tried niacin and that it had not worked, an outright lie, and that niacin would "fry his brain," another lie. Niacin might slightly increase vasodilation of the meninges of the brain, but generally does not flush the internal organs as it is a cutaneous vasokilation. The professor cruelly told this father that if he insisted on trying the niacin, they would discharge the boy, but he was too psychotic to be cared for at home.

The physician returned home very depressed, but also angry. He told his wife he was determined to start their son on the niacin. He suggested to her that they make jam sandwiches, which their son loved, each containing the niacin, ground up. The niacin could be spread on the bread and covered with jam. However, his wife was afraid and refused to do so; nevertheless, the doctor himself visited his son every afternoon, took him for a walk, and fed him the niacin-reinforced jam sandwiches. After about three or four weeks, his son said, "Daddy, every time I eat the sandwiches I turn red." The father became concerned that the boy would tell his psychiatrist and thereafter gave him niacinamide instead. Twelve weeks after starting him on the vitamin B-3, the boy said, "Daddy, I want to go home." His father discharged him. He remained on niacinamide for 18 months, and completed high school in the U.S. top 5 percentile.

Having done so well, his father then asked me if he should still continue on the niacinamide. I suggested he discontinue as a test. Six months later he began to relapse. He was again started on niacinamide, but after one month was no better. I then suggested he start on penicillamine for a few weeks, after which he made a complete recovery and has stayed on the vitamin thereafter. He graduated from university, became a physician, later a specialist, and has been working in research.

For a long time, I have been fascinated by how ideas spread from person to person. This young patient's recovery was one of the factors which alerted Linus Pauling to our use of high doses of vitamin B-3 for treating schizophrenia. The boy's recovery was considered miraculous to the small community in which his family lived. Another schizophrenic lived in the same community, and she had failed to respond to all the best treatment given to her in California, by the best therapists her desperate parents could find. When they heard about the doctor's son, they contacted me. Eventually she arrived in Saskatoon at University Hospital. There I gave her a series of ECT and started her on niacin. One month later she was well and returned home.

At that time, our book *How To Live with Schizophrenia* had just been published. Because of her recovery, this girl's father became devoted to the cause of using vitamins. He decided to approach each physician in their community and leave the book with them, hoping they would become interested. Only one was a psychiatrist, and he left a copy of the book with her. Some time later, Dr and Mrs Linus Pauling were visiting the home of the psychiatrist when Dr Pauling spotted the book on her coffee table. He borrowed it and by morning had read it through.

Dr Pauling became very interested and began to search the literature. He was not deterred by physicians who told him our work had been disproven, as he could find no negative published reports. In his own report in *Science* on "Orthomolecular Psychiatry," Dr Pauling became the most important advocate of our course of diagnosis and treatment. Since then Dr Pauling and I have often collaborated in the cause of advancing orthomolecular medicine — in research such as our study of *Vitamin C and Cancer* and in controversies with the established medical community.

The second case was started on niacin, 3 grams daily, in 1960 when she was seven years old. Annie's mother was a chronic backward schizophrenic from a mental hospital in Baltimore. She had been through a large number of New York state hospitals. Indeed, Annie was born in one of these hospitals; her mother, on one of her passes from hospital, had seduced a sailor. After Annie was born, she was adopted by her grandfather and his second wife. This couple was friendly with Mr. Bill W., co-founder of Alcoholics Anonymous. Dr Osmond and I were close friends of Bill's and and had shared with each other information about our work and his work in A.A. Annie was diagnosed mentally retarded, and the adoptive parents were advised to send her to a special school for the retarded. (In 1960 these older terms such as retarded, etc., were still in common use.) Bill W. asked me if I would see Annie on my next visit to New York. Her parents told me she could not learn and that she was developing serious behavioral problems. I advised them to start her on niacinamide 3 grams per day.

Two years later, Bill once more asked me to see Annie. Her parents were very discouraged because they had seen no change in her. By then I had had only limited experience with children. I could only hope that if they were patient, she would eventually respond. The following year she began to get better. She went through the regular school system, went on the college, graduated on the Dean's list, and became a teacher. Several years ago I received a letter from her mother, inviting me to Annie's wedding in Washington, D.C. I had seen Annie only twice as a child and once later on during her late teens. She was still well in 1997.

These two examples of the outcome of treatment over many years are very special to me because they were among the first children so treated. Since then, this experience has been confirmed on over 1500 children, most of whom responded; the failures simply did not stay on the program long enough. A full account of my work with children is available in my book *Dr Hoffer's A,B,C of Natural Nutrition for Children*.

These two cases also placed orthomolecular psychiatry in the spotlight by association with such high-profile and controversial advocates as Linus Pauling and Bill W. The battle for acceptance has lasted over forty years.

CONTROVERSY

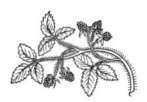

The Politics of Ideas

American Psychiatric Association

Medical Establishment

The New Medical Paradigm

THE POLITICS OF IDEAS

Controversy is part of the history of medicine and essential if medicine is to continue to improve or advance. New ideas will always challenge established practice: research and experience will prove some new ideas wrong, some right, some pernicious, some promising. I soon found myself and my colleagues entangled in such controversy following a report I wrote on the two children from California I treated for schizophrenia with vitamin B-3. Having two-time Nobel Peace Prize Winner Linus Pauling at our side proved to be both a comfort and a goad as Dr Osmond and I confronted the negative and decidedly undemocratic and unscientific response from the American Psychiatric Association and the medical establishment to our research.

American Psychiatric Association

The response to vitamin B-3 by the two California patients aroused considerable interest, and within a short time I had a chance to treat a few more. I published a little paper in 1967 in the *Journal of Schizophrenia* which I called "Five California Schizophrenics." These patients all shared four attributes: they were from California, they had failed to respond to standard treatment, I treated them for their disease, and they were greatly improved. Four of the patients became normal and one became much better.

I had hoped the title of the paper would arouse the interest of American psychiatrists so they would repeat the treatment on their own patients. The consequences of this report were totally surprising. There was no attempt to repeat our work, but it spurred the American psychiatrists into a serious attempt to prevent us from publishing any more vitamin B-3 reports. Perhaps my conclusion was too provocative when I wrote, "Every patient had been diagnosed and treated in the best psychiatric centers in California and elsewhere, and not one had responded to psychoanalysis and tranquilizers. In other words those five had already proven they were not going to respond spontaneously."

A few years after this report was published, I received a letter from the American Psychiatric Association. I was at that time a Fellow and had been a member for some time. (One year the APA elected a Canadian to be its president, Ewen Cameron, professor of psychiatry at McGill University. For political reasons they wanted to induct a good Canadian representation into their fellowship ranks. I was one of the Canadians invited to join. There was no advantage to me but the annual dues were heavier.) The letter from the APA stated that Dr Osmond and I had been accused of promoting unorthodox treatment for schizophrenia. The letter demanded we cease and desist.

I then read the constitution of the APA and its by-laws for the first time. I concluded the Board of the APA had not followed its own by-laws. They should have placed the complaint against us before their Committee on Ethics, who would call upon us to get our views. They would then, if they saw the need to do so, send a recommendation to the Board, who would subsequently act. We had been given the mildest possible reprimand, a slap on the wrist, but in failing to follow their own by-laws the APA had committed an unconstitutional act.

I promptly wrote back, bringing this to their attention and demanding that the matter should be placed before the appropriate committee. I also requested to know the names of the psychiatrists who had made the complaint and the exact charges against us. The irony of the situation was that, as a Canadian, the APA had no jurisdiction over me and could not prevent me from practicing as I wished. After many months of corresponding, the APA arranged for us to meet with their committee in Washington, D.C., in 1972. They also informed us the complaint arose from my paper, "Five California Schizophrenics," and had come from one or more California psychiatrists, who never were identified. This also contravened APA by-laws because, according to U.S. law, the accused have the right to know who their accusers are.

Dr Osmond and I nevertheless arranged to meet in Washington the day before the hearing. I had planned to spend the previous week in New York where I was to tape five sessions of the popular television show, "For Women Only." After Washington I was to go to San Juan to speak to the National Cancer Institute meeting on the fallacies of the double-blind controlled experiment. Thus scheduling was critical. Two days before I left for New York, I received a wire from the APA. They could not meet us on the day originally set but would meet the following day. This was impossible for us, as I was leaving for San Juan. I looked upon this as another example of harassment. After talking to Dr Osmond, I wired back that the new day they had selected was impossible, that we were holding them to the original date, and that we would be there at APA headquarters at 9 a.m. as previously arranged, whether they were there or not. To our relief they were all there.

The meeting turned into a farce. As far as I could tell, not a single member had read any of our papers and their knowledge of vitamins was almost nil. After our introduction, their legal advisor asked our permission to tape the conversation. Their lawyer asked me a very simple question, "Are you the A. Hoffer who wrote 'Five California Schizophrenics'"? I agreed that I was that A. Hoffer. He then asked me the same question two more times. By that time I was irritated and annoyed. After that formality, I announced that although Dr Osmond and I were there, we did not accept the right of their committee to judge our treatment. It was not a matter of ethics, I said. It was more properly a matter for their Committee on Science. They knew I was angry and tried to mollify us by practicing psychiatric wiles used on irritable patients. They assured us they were there under two hats: one hat they wore for the Committee on Ethics, and the other as colleagues of ours, sincerely interested in hearing about our work. I retorted that we would be pleased to spend all day talking about our work to our colleagues, but we did not accept their hat for the Committee on Ethics.

Then they made a statement I had anticipated. They said that Dr Nathan Kline had tried to confirm our work and had failed. Because of their ignorance of vitamins, they confused vitamin B-3, which was the subject of the charge, with its coenzyme, nicotinamide adenine dinucleotide, which Kline had tested using a product which was different from the one we used. I had written to Kline requesting him to confirm that he had never tried vitamin B-3, and he promptly sent me the letter. As soon as the charge was levelled against us at the meeting, I pulled out Dr Kline's letter and read it to them. The rest of the morning Dr Osmond and I discussed our controlled experiments and our clinical data.

At 11:45 a.m. the committee chairman announced they would leave us for a few moments while they deliberated. Thirty minutes later they returned; the committee had not been able to reach a decision. They said they would write to us with their decision in a few days. We have not yet received their letter. It was good politics not to reach any conclusion. Had they found us guilty, we would have appealed and received a lot more publicity. Had they sent us a letter stating they had found no substantiation of the charges against us, we could have used that document in our public presentations. We could have answered any critics by simply saying that the APA found our work to be ethical. Shortly after we returned from Washington, I resigned my fellowship from the APA, declaring I could not tolerate their behavior and attitude toward our research, and I would contribute no more money (annual dues) to enable them to attack us.

But the APA did succeed in an effort to discredit our

work a year later in 1973 with their "Task Force 7: Report on Megavitamins and Orthomolecular Therapy in Psychiatry." This report apparently was prompted by our meeting with the APA and perhaps by our relationship with JD, a labor leader in California, the first to introduce psychiatric treatment in a health clinic for union members (Local 770). The APA was then in a very expansive mood and firmly believed that, given a chance, every person ought to be psychoanalyzed, including presidents, governors, legislators, and more; this move by JD's union represented a major advance in their design to psychiatrize the world.

Unfortunately, JD's daughter became schizophrenic and received psychoanalytic treatment from the psychiatrist working at their clinic. She did not get well. JD was so upset over his daughter's illness and the lack of response that he began to read what he could. He obtained a biochemical text book and began to read it very slowly and painfully. He could not understand most of the words. Each day he would take these underlined words, one page per day, give them to his secretary, who would look them up in a medical dictionary and write out the definition. Half way through this text he ran across a section on pellagra and niacin. He suddenly realized that the symptoms described for pellagra were almost identical with his daughter's. He discussed this with the chief of his clinic, a internist, who told him about our work in Canada. JD promptly called me, and we discussed his daughter's illness.

In spite of my assurance about the safety of niacin therapy, JD was fearful. He decided to take niacin himself for one month: if he survived, he would then give it to his daughter. He survived, and his daughter recovered. JD now was fired with enthusiasm because he saw a new treatment for members of his union with similar problems. Early in 1971 JD promoted a meeting in Los Angeles. Several of my colleagues and I presented our findings. A medical student who had recovered from schizophrenia under my care by taking niacin (and who now practices orthomolecular psychiatry) came to the meeting and outlined his illness and recovery. The APA heard about this meeting and commissioned Dr Morris Lipton to contact JD to request that he be permitted also to appear on the platform. JD checked with me and I agreed that Lipton would be given the same time as the rest of us. I had not heard about him before but felt that there was no need to shut out criticism. The hall was full with about 1500 attending.

Before the meeting started, Dr Ross MacLean, chairman of the meeting, told me that Lipton had approached him to demand three times as much time since he was only one against the rest of us. This was not granted. During his talk he stated (1) that he had never used megavitamin therapy; (2) that he did not treat schizophrenic patients; and (3) that because he had been a graduate student in Wisconsin in the same department where Dr Elvehjem had proved niacin was vitamin B-3, this made him an expert on the vitamin. Then he launched a savage attack on orthomolecular theory and practice. Later, Lipton was appointed chairman of the "APA Task Force 7: Report on Megavitamins and Orthomolecular Therapy in Psychiatry" and wrote the major recommendations discrediting our work based on his address that day. After the meeting JD sent me a copy of the text Lipton had prepared with the assistance of his colleague Dr F.J. Kane at the North Carolina Department of Psychiatry; the final APA Task Force report was merely an elaboration of the paper he read at that meeting in Los Angeles. Thereafter psychiatrists, including the Canadian Psychiatric Association, looked upon this as the gospel since they could not believe that an official document put forth by a major professional organization could be full of deceit and lies.

I think these two episodes were the factors that led the APA to launch their attack. They knew what they were going to find and they decided to promote it as vigorously as possible. They appointed a committee of whom most were dedicated opponents of megavitamin therapy. Besides chairman Dr Morris Lipton and Dr F.J. Kane, Dr Loren E. Mosher, head of the Center for Studies of Schizophrenia, National Institute for Mental Health, Washington, D.C., did not believe that there was such a disease as schizophrenia, and if it did exist, the only treatment was psychotherapy following Dr R.D. Laing approach, in special homes where they would be treated with love and more love. (No one ever recovered on this kind of love.) His colleague at the NIMH and fellow Task Force member Dr J. Levine shared a similar faith in Laing's approach. Task Force member Dr Thomas Ban had previously attempted to discredit our work in 1966 when he was commissioned by the Canadian Mental Health Association to settle the matter of "Hoffer's megavitamin claims once and for all." Ban was well known for his studies with tranquilizers and received much of his income from sources interested in promoting tranquilizers for treatment of schizophrenia.

The 54-page Task Force report begins by stating "we shall examine carefully and critically the claims, the supporting evidence, the theoretical basis and the contrary evidence in detail." The report concludes that "the credibility of the megavitamin proponents is low" before issuing the following warning: "Under these circumstances this Task Force considers the massive publicity they promulgate via radio, the lay press and popular books, using catch phrases which are really misnomers like 'megavitamin therapy' and 'orthomolecular treatment,' to be deplorable."

In 1976 Dr Osmond and I published a 120-page reply to this report, still available from the Canadian Schizophrenia Foundation. The APA Task Force report is out of print. "Our criticism of the committee and their report," we wrote, "is that: (1) The committee was in composition biased, failing to contain anyone who was familiar by personal experience with orthomolecular therapy. (2) The procedure used by the committee failed to ensure any objectivity or fairness, for (i) they did not obtain any evidence from anyone using orthomolecular therapy; and (ii) they selectively examined the literature using the rule that any double-blind study or allegedly double-blind study (even if it were not like the Wittenborn and Ban studies) was evidence if it yielded negative results while conversely no clinical study if positive was scientific. The four original double blinds studies from Saskatchewan were suspect since we did them, so were not evidence. (3) The report is characterized by falsehoods, direct and by inference, by biased statement, by the use of brief sentences taken out of context, by omissions which always favored the committee's view. (4) The report was written in order to bolster the committee's negative conclusions.

"Unfortunately, the committee was correct in their assumption that most psychiatrists who read their report would accept it at face value and would not check their references. The report has had a pernicious effect in dampening interest in orthomolecular psychiatry. While this will not hurt any orthomolecular psychiatrists, it will condemn hundreds of thousands of patients to a lifetime of tranquilized chronicity.

"Community psychiatry, which is essentially an expensive system for delivering tranquilizers to chronic patients in various shelters, is coming more and more into disfavor. Psychiatrists are sinking lower and lower in both public esteem and in the esteem of their non-psychiatric medical colleagues. The printing and distribution by the APA of a report so bigoted and biased as the Task Force Report can serve only to drive the psychiatric profession lower in public esteem." What we wrote in 1976 was prescient, except that today the streets have become the main hospital for chronic patients and it is much more difficult to deliver these drugs to patients with no permanent home.

Dr Linus Pauling examined this report at length and wrote, "The APA task force report on Megavitamin and Orthomolecular Therapy in Psychiatry discusses vitamins in a very limited way (niacin only) and deals with only one of two aspects of the theory. Its arguments are in part faulty and its conclusions are unjustified."

In retrospect, I think one of our main problems was that the results were too good and psychiatrists accustomed only to the impact of tranquilizers could not believe that vitamins could be so effective. Psychiatry is brainwashed by the numerous and beautiful advertisements present in all the medical journals. In some journals 70 percent of their pages are advertisements. Reading these journals and these advertisements is the post graduate education of most psychiatrists. The emphasis on drug treatments is reinforced by the sales people of the drug companies. They are pleasant, attractive, knowledgeable promoters willing to leave samples and valuable information, all about their drugs. (When they visit me, as they do regularly, I teach them about the value of orthomolecular therapy.)

Despite our arguments and proof, established medical opinion sided with the APA and we soon found ourselves unable to publish in many medical journals. In my opinion, the APA was responsible for slowing down the acceptance of megavitamin therapy by twenty years. How many millions of schizophrenic patients have been condemned to permanent illness by this action of the APA?

Medical Establishment

Naive physicians have, over the years, tried to destroy our claims by dismissing them with the simplistic question, "If the results are so good, why isn't every psychiatrist practicing this way?" They assume that every physician is burning with desire to use the latest advances in medicine to benefit their patients. In fact, most physicians are burning with a quite different desire — to practice in such a way that they will not be attacked by their own regulatory bodies, like the colleges of physicians and surgeons, and also to avoid being attacked in court by patients or their families. The surest way of avoiding censure from colleagues is to do what they are doing; that is, practicing what they were taught in medical school and in their graduate training.

The enslavement by old ideas and the dread of new experiences is an ancient characteristic of humankind. Moses led the Israelites out of Egypt to the Promised Land. The whole trip, even on foot, should have taken several weeks. So why did it take forty years? This must have been one of the most circuitous journeys in history, to walk the desert in huge circles, edging ever closer to Palestine. This was not due to poor navigation. According to the Bible, Moses realized that he could not hope to prevail over the natives of Palestine with a group of people who had been born in slavery; they knew no other way of life. He concluded he would need two generations of men and women born in freedom in the desert before they would have the vigor and spirit to undertake the task of conquering the Promised Land. He needed two generations of freedom to convert slaves into free men and women. Physicians, too, need two generations of freedom from old theories and practices.

Several years ago I gave a twenty minute address to the Nutrition Committee of the New York State Medical Association. About twenty five people were there. The chairperson was sympathetic and I had a sympathetic audience. However, one young man who had a professorial air about him fell asleep as soon as I started my presentation. He awakened promptly just before I finished. I had concluded he was an academic with a lot of exposure to new ideas, which he dealt with by not listening. During the question period, he hit me with what he considered a devastating criticism. I had heard this one very frequently over the years. He said, "Dr Hoffer, if your treatment is so good, why isn't every doctor using it?" I replied by telling him about Moses and two generations in the desert, adding that when two generations of doctors enslaved by their medical schools had passed on, our treatment would be accepted. Our starting date was 1957 when we first published our vitamin B-3 treatment paper. My critic quickly subsided while the other members of the audience smiled, but he did remain awake.

The standard medical journals are closed to innovative medical researchers and the new material often cannot be published. Since these are the only journals read by physicians, they have no chance to become aware of the data — or of the conflict of ideas generated by it. But derogatory material, no matter how biased or false, is rapidly published in the same journals. Generally editors are less biased and more open to new ideas than are the reviewers or referees to whom they send manuscripts for their opinion. Editors in so-called refereed journals will select several reviewers who will eventually give their opinion whether or not an article should be published. The manuscript is sent to experts in the field, presumably because they are most familiar with the field. But since they are experts in the field, they are much less likely to allow papers to be published which run counter to their own ideas. A paper describing the use of vitamins will be rejected by such a committee whose members "know" vitamins cannot be helpful. Only a paper written by a person of enormous professional stature, from a highly respected institution, is likely to be accepted if the ideas are different. But the resistance toward the new idea may be so strong, even scientists of the stature of Linus Pauling will find their manuscripts rejected. Thus, orthomolecular papers have been rejected so frequently that standard journals no longer receive any of these manuscripts.

In sharp contrast, papers attacking orthomolecular concepts appear to sail right through editorial committees.

For this reason, a very poor study was published in the *Journal of the American Medical Association* which claimed in the title and in the conclusion that ascorbic acid destroyed vitamin B-12 and could cause pernicious anemia. However, the data in the body of the paper did not support this conclusion. The journal of the AMA refused to publish even one letter pointing out this error to them. Another example is a paper published in *The New England Journal of Medicine* where the authors claimed: (1) they had repeated exactly studies previously reported by Drs E. Cameron and L. Pauling; and (2) that they could not confirm these original studies. In fact, their first claim was not true and therefore their conclusion was irrelevant. *The New England Journal of Medicine* refused to publish a rebuttal written by Dr Pauling.

Physicians who do embrace or even entertain new ideas are often censured, up to and including loss of license to practice, but this step is rarely necessary, as the simple threat this can happen will keep most doctors in line, away from orthomolecular medicine. Many physicians have lost their license to practice. They were skillful, innovative physicians who helped patients recover, in many cases when no previous treatment had helped. One of the charges against one of my colleagues was that he gave his patients intravenous ascorbic acid. Another charge was that he had his patients do the Hoffer-Osmond Diagnostic (HOD) test.

Physicians have also been excommunicated by their colleagues. Many years ago, I received a letter from a psychiatrist who described how happy he was with the results he was getting using vitamin B-3. I wrote back to him, requesting his permission to give his name to patients in his area who were seeking doctors who would use vitamin B-3. Six months later he wrote again, requesting that I not give out his name anymore. He told me the results he was seeing were as good as before, but if he continued to use vitamin B-3 his life would be destroyed in his city. He said his psychiatric colleagues and friends would no longer speak to him, and that if he did not stop using this treatment, he would lose his hospital privileges. He added he could only continue if he transplanted his family to a new area, and that he was too well established to make such a drastic move.

Another psychiatrist was forced to move to a different city, where he became a successful orthomolecular psychiatrist. A director of psychiatric research at a state hospital near San Francisco told me he would love to start therapeutic trials with vitamin B-3, but that if he did, he would be fired, and any chance of continuing his career in California would be lost to him forever.

THE NEW MEDICAL PARADIGM

The methods used to prevent new paradigms from gaining acceptance are very interesting, and they must be exposed to public view if we are ever to shorten the interval between discovery and general application. This huge lag between discovery and acceptance is very costly to society, as it prevents good treatments from being used and denies millions of patients the benefit of treatment. The usual reaction of doctors is to claim that the present system prevents bad treatments from being introduced. In fact it does not, for the acceptability of new ideas depends very much on their source. A good idea from Harvard Medical School will receive more serious attention than the same idea from South Dakota or Saskatchewan. The politics of ideas are much more influential in the acceptance of a new treatment than are its merits.

Medicine is a very conservative profession when it is confronted by major changes in theory and practice. Major clashes in theory and practice are, in reality, clashes between old and new paradigms or ways of seeing the world

— or practicing medicine. In response to such an assault, the profession closes ranks and defends itself with every means at its disposal. Tactics include denial, ostracism, censure, and dismissal.

Denial that a new paradigm has any scientific merit is the simplest reaction. Denial is first practiced by ignoring the claims put forward by the new paradigm. Later there is a direct attack upon the new paradigm by the leaders of the profession. The counterattack will take many forms; for example, they will state that the new claims have not been established scientifically, that the case histories of patient recoveries are of no value because they are anecdotal, and that the onus is on the proponents of new treatments to prove their claims using the scientific method. The scientific method, in modern terms, means prospective double-blind controlled experiments. Critics will concede some individual patients are helped, but in the same breath will maintain this does not constitute proof because it is merely anecdotal. Only double-blind controlled experiments are scientific, they claim.

In fact, this is more a statement of faith than a scientific principle. It is true that a treatment is of no value if it does not change the natural history of a disease. If penicillin, when it was introduced, cured 30 percent of all cases of pneumonia, and if without treatment, there was a 30 percent survival, then one could assume it was not effective. Therefore, one must know the natural history of diseases, although groups of patients will vary with location, time, etc. Thus, Doctor A may find 50 percent of the patients given drug A will respond, while Doctor B may find that only 30 percent do. This is a natural variation.

To help establish the natural recovery rate, one must work with two groups: one group is kept as a control, the other is treated. If the treated group is a lot better, one can conclude the treatment was effective. This principle is well established in all biological research, from growing crops to treating animals. The double-blind controlled experiment goes one step further by introducing blindness into the study: neither patient nor the evaluators of the treatment know whether active drug or no drug (placebo) has been given. This is based on the hypothesis that this type of experiment will remove the effect of faith and hope from the patient, and bias from the evaluator. It is a pious hope, sanctified by slavish adherence to the method. In fact, I have not been able to find a single scientific report that has tested this theory; there are no experiments which prove the validity of this hypothesis. But to question the hypothesis creates anger and hostility; followers of this theory refuse to believe the emperor has no clothes. Any clinical study not done double-blind is decreed to be anecdotal. This, to a pure psychiatric research scientist, is almost as bad as raping one's patient. The word 'anecdotal' is not a bad one. It means an interesting history. The major difference between a purely anecdotal study and a double-blind anecdotal study is that in the latter the history is deficient, since it is not known what drug the patient has been on.

There has been an encouraging reaction against deriding anecdotal studies. Clinicians are developing N = 1 studies; i.e., either drug or placebo is given serially to one patient and the results are recorded. They are even using the word anecdote in the title of their papers and then writing their reports as if their conclusions were as relevant as they would be if they had been double-blind studies. The proper reply to a critic who throws the word anecdotal at you is to ask why they are so impressed with the double-blind hypothesis, which has as yet not been tested rigorously by any proper experiment.

Every one of these tactics arises from the enslavement of the medical profession to the currently accepted theory and practice of their profession. This is why it has taken forty years for many major medical discoveries to come into general use. This gap between discovery and general application has applied to major discoveries, including the discovery of the circulation of blood, the germ theory of disease, the use of vitamins in treating deficiency diseases, cardiac catheterization, the use of electrocardiograms and electroencephalograms, and more.

Nor is it true that the present system has protected us against new treatment ideas later found to be ineffective. I cannot think of a single idea in psychiatry which was kept out of practice by controlled studies. Psychoanalysis, the least effective treatment of all, is still with us after 100 years. The system did not protect us from that. Every treatment ever introduced in psychiatry has been used until it was supplanted by one which was more effective and less dangerous — or perhaps merely different.

For schizophrenics, the most dangerous treatment of all was to warehouse them in terrible institutions for their lifetime. In time, this was replaced by insulin coma therapy and more humane care. Insulin coma was, in turn, replaced by electroconvulsive therapy, which is no longer needed as frequently but still plays a limited role. Tranquilizers came in relatively quickly but there were special circumstances, chiefly that they are patented and it profited pharmaceutical companies to re-educate the medical profession. This was done by spending millions of dollars each year on advertising, meetings, seminars, and drug salesmen. Tranquilizers, incidentally, were the first patented drugs sold by pharmaceutical companies to be used in psychiatry. There was also enormous pressure from a group of forty senators and congressmen in Washington to vanquish the psychoanalytic bias of the National Institutes of Mental Health and allow them to sponsor tranquilizer studies. From a scientific point of view, the numerous double-blind controlled studies costing millions of dollars were not necessary, since no information was gained. The studies served mainly to persuade psychiatrists, especially at medical schools, to start using these drugs.

The only new progress in the so-called tranquilizer decades (1955 to 1991) has been the development of new tranquilizers and the refinement of ways of getting them into patients. We know more about probable mechanisms than before, but no more about their clinical use. However, even with enormous pressure from drug companies, even with the clear and dramatic effect of tranquilizers, and even with half the content of psychiatric journals devoted to tranquilizer studies, it still took from 1954 to about 1965 before they were finally "in."

Although vitamin and nutrient therapy developed over the same period as tranquilizer therapy, widespread acceptance by the public and the medical profession did not begin until the early 1990s. One of the first signs of an acceptance of this new medical paradigm was an article published in the *New York Times,* March 10, 1992 under the headline "Vitamins Win Support as Potent Agents of Health." The *Times* had not been as enthusiastic a decade earlier when the paper commissioned a freelance reporter to attend a meeting of the Huxley Institute of Biosocial Research in New York. I was then president of HIBS. After the two-day meeting, the reporter approached me for an interview, which he prefaced by telling me that he had expected to encounter a bunch of quacks and kooks at this meeting, but instead met a group of bona fide medical doctors and researchers of the highest order and sobriety reporting on their findings. I initially refused to spend any time with him when he told me he was from the *Times,* suspecting they would not publish anything favorable about our work since the paper was then clearly in the camp of the medical 'profession'. He then assured me he had never had an article rejected by his editors, and with that assurance I spent about six hours with him outlining the history and efficacy of orthomolecular medicine. However, the report never appeared.

Time Magazine, April 6, 1992, was next with their cover story "The Real Power of Vitamins," subtitled "New

Research Shows They May Help Fight Cancer, Heart Disease and the Ravages of Aging" — all claims that Linus Pauling, Irwin Stone, Humphry Osmond, my other colleagues, and I had made years before. The *Time* report concluded: "Vitamins promise to continue to unfold as one of the great and hopeful health stories of our day." *The Medical Post*, April 23, 1992, reported that vitamin C may lower heart disease risk, and on May 8, 1992 the *New York Times* again reported, "Vitamin C Linked to Heart Benefit: It May also Help Prevent an Early Death from Other Disease." *Newsweek* finally joined ranks May 8, 1992 with their story: "Live Longer with Vitamin C."

The Harvard Health Letter, *Johns Hopkins Medical Letter*, and the *Diet-Heart Newsletter* all reported similar stories to their audience of health professionals. And the medical profession was alerted to the arrival of this new paradigm by the *New England Journal of Medicine* in a 1993 study which reported that in 1990 more Americans consulted alternative practitioners than all U.S. primary care physicians, 425 million visits versus 388 million. The social demographic group who consulted these alternative practitioners were non-black, ranging in age from 25 to 49 years, with relatively more education and higher incomes. They consulted them for chronic conditions. Twelve percent of this group sought megavitamin therapy — 51 million visits were devoted to this form of orthomolecular therapy. The authors advised the profession should ascertain from their patients information about their use of alternative therapies, but I doubt this will be forthcoming since most patients who have consulted me are still not willing to discuss it with their doctors because of the negative reactions they have heard in the past. The article concluded that "medical schools should include information about unconventional therapies and the clinical social sciences (anthropology and sociology) in their curriculums. The newly established National Institutes of Health Office for the Study of Unconventional Medical Practices should help promote scholarly research and education in this area."

I would add that much of this scholarly and scientific research already exists in the pages of alternative medicine publications such as the *Journal of Orthomolecular Medicine*. The pioneering work we began in Saskatchewan in the early 1950s seems to be on the verge of becoming the medical paradigm of the next century.

APPENDIX ONE

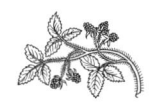

HOD Test Questionnaire

A. Hoffer, PhD, MD

H. Osmond, MD

HOD TEST QUESTIONNAIRE

This inventory consists of numbered statements. Read each statement and answer it either True or False according to how well it describes what is happening to you.

You are to put your answers on the answer sheet. Look at the example of the answer sheet shown at the right. If the statement is True as applied to you, draw a circle around the T opposite the number of that statement on the answer sheet. (See item number 26 at the right.) If, for example, statement number 37 is False as applied to you, draw a circle around the F opposite number 37 on the answer sheet. (See number 37 in the above example.)

Example of how to record an answer
26. (T) F
37. T (F)

Answer every statement.

Each statement in this questionnaire is numbered, but the numbers are not arranged in consecutive order. The order of the numbers in the booklet and on the answer sheet, however, are the same. In marking your answers on the answer sheet, be sure that the number of the statement in the booklet is the same as the number you are answering on the answer sheet. Erase any answer you wish to change. Do not make any marks on this questionnaire.

Remember, answer every statement as it applies to you, and be sure that the number of each statement in the booklet is the same number you are answering on the answer sheet.

NOW GO AHEAD.

47. Some foods which never tasted funny before do so now.
143. Most people hate me.
68. There are some people trying to do me harm.
61. I can no longer smell perfumes as well as I used to.
60. I sweat much more now than when I used to.

59. My body odor is now much more unpleasant.
134. People interfere with my body to harm me.
66. My mind is racing away from me.
81. People are watching me.
73. At times when I come into a new situation, I feel strongly the situation is a repeat of one that happened before.

10. Sometimes I have visions of animals or scenes.
70. I have a mission in life given to me by God.
2. People's faces seem to change in size as I watch them.
86. A dress is like a glove because they belong to women rather than because they are articles of clothing.
5. People watch me all the time.

46. I sometimes feel strange vibrations shivering through me.
15. When I look at people they seem strange.
22. Sometimes when I watch TV the picture looks very strange.
141. I don't like meeting people — you can't trust anyone now.
117. My hands or feet sometimes feel far away.

107. Life seems entirely hopeless.
106. I usually feel miserable and blue.
51. Water now has funny tastes.

121. I often hear my thoughts inside my head.
 92. An axe is like a saw because they have handles rather than because they are tools.

110. I have to be on my guard with friends.
 82. A cow is like a horse because they are both in North America, not because they are both animals.
 78. My thinking gets all mixed up when I have to act quickly.
126. Other people's cigarette smoke smells strange — like a gas.
 50. I have more difficulty tasting foods now.

 49. Foods taste flat and lifeless.
  7. Most people have halos (areas of brightness) around their heads.
 35. I have often felt that there was another voice in my head.
 31. I now have more trouble hearing people.
140. I get more frightened now when I am driven in a car by others.

  6. I feel rays of energy upon me.
 28. I sometimes feel that I have left my body.
  1. People's faces sometimes pulsate as I watch them.
123. I hear my own thoughts as clearly as if they were a voice.
109. I am often misunderstood by people.

 45. I now have trouble feeling hot or cold things.
 27. My hands or feet sometimes seem much too large for me.
 39. I sometimes have sensations of crawly things under my skin.
 64. At times my ideas disappear for a few moments and then reappear.

88. A pen is like a pencil because they are like sticks, rather than because they are used for writing.

85. A chair is like a table because they are usually used together rather than because they both have four legs.
84. A chair is like a table because they have four legs, not because they are usually used together.
19. Sometimes the world becomes very bright as I look at it.
133. Many people know that I have a mission in life.
80. Strange people or places frighten me.

21. Sometimes when I read the words begin to look funny — they move around or grow faint.
52. I can no longer tell how much time has gone by.
127. The world has become timeless for me.
116. I often become scared of sudden movements or noises at night.
43. I sometimes feel my bowels are dead.

58. My body odor is much more noticeable than it once was.
14. When I look at things like tables and chairs they seem strange.
37. I have heard voices coming from radio, television, or tape recorders talking about me.
137. People interfere with my mind to help me.
11. Sometimes I have visions of God or of Christ.

34. I often hear or have heard voices talking about or to me.
25. Pictures appear to be alive and to breathe.
145. I am not sure who I am.
138. I know that most people expect a great deal of me.
41. Some of my organs feel dead.

30. My sense of hearing is now more sensitive than it ever has been.
  4. People watch me a lot more than they used to.
108. I am very painfully shy.
 20. Sometimes the world becomes very dim as I look at it.
114. I am constantly keyed up and jittery.

 54. Some days move by so quickly it seems only minutes have gone by.
  3. People's eyes seem very piercing and frightening.
103. I very often suffer from severe nervous exhaustion.
 36. I have often heard strange sounds, e.g. laughing which frightens me.
125. Cigarettes taste queer now.

 32. I often have singing noises in my ears.
 42. I sometimes feel my stomach is dead.
124. My bones often feel soft.
 38. My sense of touch has now become very keen.
  9. Sometimes I have visions of people during the day when my eyes are open.

100. A fly is like a tree because they both require humans rather than because they are living things.
 17. Now and then when I'd look in the mirror my face changes and seems different.
  8. Sometimes I have visions of people when I close my eyes.
 16. Often when I look at people they seem to be like someone else.
 33. I often hear or have heard voices.

111. Very often friends irritate me.
 40. I sometimes feel rays of electricity shooting through me.
101. A fly is like a tree because they both are living

things rather than because they both require humans.
71. At times some other people can read my mind.
120. When I am driving in a car objects and people change shape very quickly. They didn't used to.

75. I am now much more forgetful.
56. I have much more trouble getting my work done on time.
115. Sudden noises make me jump or shake badly.
55. I have much more trouble keeping appointments.
90. An orange is like a banana because they both have skins rather than because they are fruit.

98. Praise is like punishment because they both start with p rather than because they are given to people.
132. People are often envious of me.
62. Foods smell funny now.
136. People interfere with my mind to harm me.
69. There is some plot against me.

76. I now am sick.
118. My hands or feet often look very small now.
94. The eye is like the ear because they are on the head rather than because they are sense organs.
89. A pen is like a pencil because they are both used for writing rather than because they both are like sticks.
113. I am often very shaky.

104. I very often have great difficulty falling asleep at night.
48. I can taste bitter things in some foods like poison.
130. People look as if they were dead now.
112. My family irritates me very much.

139. Lately I often get frightened when driving myself in a car.

13. Sometimes I feel very unreal.
119. Cars seem to move very quickly now. I can't be sure where they are.
23. Sometimes I feel there is a fog or mist shutting me away from the world.
91. An orange is like a banana because they are fruit, not because they both have skins
93. An axe is like a saw because they are tools rather than because they have handles.

87. A dress is like a glove because they are articles of clothing rather than because they are owned by women.
95. The eye is like the ear because they are sense organs rather than because they are on the head.
102. I very often am very tired.
53. The days seem to go by very slowly.
24. Sometimes objects pulsate when I look at them.

129. Other people smell strange.
44. I sometimes feel I am being pinched by unseen things.
18. My body now and then seems to be altered — too big or too small, out of proportion.
135. People interfere with my body to help me.
122. I often hear my own thoughts outside my head.

57. Things smell very funny now.
144. I find that past, present and future seem all muddled up.
12. Sometimes the world seems unreal.
105. I usually feel alone and sad at a party.
131. I feel as if I am dead.

29. I often feel I have left my body.
26. I often see sparks or spots of light floating before me.
97. Air is like water because they are needed for life rather than because they are both cold.
99. Praise is like punishment because they are both given to people rather than because they start with the letter p.
65. I am bothered by very disturbing ideas.

83. A cow is like a horse because they are animals, not because they are in North America.
128. Time seems to have changed recently, but I am not sure how.
79. I very often get directions wrong.
72. I can read other people's minds.
77. I cannot make up my mind about things that before did not trouble me.

74. I now become easily confused.
63. At times my mind goes blank.
142. More people admire me now than ever before.
96. Air is like water because they are both cold rather than because they are needed for life.
67. At times I am aware of people talking about me.

HOD
ANSWER SHEET

Name

Sex   Age   Date

47. T F	110. T F	21. T F	32. T F	76. T F	57. T F
143. T F	82. T F	52. T F	42. T F	118. T F	144. T F
68. T F	78. T F	127. T F	124. T F	94. T F	12. T F
61. T F	126. T F	116. T F	38. T F	89. T F	105. T F
60. T F	50. T F	43. T F	9. T F	113. T F	131. T F
59. T F	49. T F	58. T F	100. T F	104. T F	29. T F
134. T F	7. T F	14. T F	17. T F	48. T F	26 T F
66. T F	35. T F	37. T F	8. T F	130. T F	97. T F
81. T F	31. T F	137. T F	16. T F	112. T F	99. T F
73. T F	140. T F	11. T F	33. T F	139. T F	65. T F
10. T F	6. T F	34. T F	111 T F	13. T F	83. TF
70. T F	28. T F	25. T F	40. T F	119. T F	128. T F
2. T F	1. T F	145. T F	101. T F	23. T F	79. T F
86. T F	123. T F	138. T F	71. T F	91. T F	72. T F
5. T F	109. T F	41. T F	120. T F	93. T F	77. T F
46. T F	45. T F	30. T F	75. T F	87. T F	74. T F
15. T F	27. T F	4. T F	56. T F	95. T F	63. T F
22. T F	39. T F	108. T F	115. T F	102. T F	142. T F
141. T F	64. T F	20. T F	55. T F	53. T F	96. T F
117. T F	88. T F	114. T F	90. T F	24. T F	67. T F
107. T F	85. T F	54. T F	98. T F	129. T F	
106. T F	84. T F	3. T F	132. T F	44. T F	
51. T F	19. T F	103. T F	62. T F	18. T F	
121. T F	133. T F	36. T F	136. T F	135. T F	
92. T F	80. T F	125. T F	69. T F	122. T F	

APPENDIX TWO

Kryptopyrroluria Test

Procedure

MEASURING KRYTOPYRROLURIA (KP) IN URINE
(2,4 dimethyl-3-ethyl pyrrole)

Urine is collected in a container containing 1 tablet of vitamin C, 500 mg. This preserves the KP.

A 2 ml urine sample is placed in a glass stoppered centrifuge tube and extracted with 4 mg of chloroform by shaking either by hand or on a Vortex shaker for about 2 minutes. After centrifugation the top aqueous layer is carefully removed and 100 to 200 mgm of anhydrous sodium sulfate is added to the chloroform and shaken briefly to remove traces of aqueous globules.

2 ml of the clear chloroform extract are placed in a clean test tube and 0.5 ml of a 1% solution of p-dimethylamino benazaldehyde (Ehrlich's reagent) in Methanol containing 5 Vol % sulfuric acid are added and shaken briefly. After 30 minutes a deep pink color will develop if KP is present. The intensity of the color is read in a spectrophotometer at 540 mu. The normal range is 0 to 20 u% — patients may read as high as 200 to 300 u%.

A standard Kryptopyrrole solution containing 1 ug to 15 ug is prepared for establishing a standard curve.

Notes:
1. The Ehrlich's reagent is prepared once weekly and it is stored in a brown bottle.
2. Kryptopyrrole is a liquid obtained in an ampule from Aldrich Chemical Company, and is very sensitive to air. Once the ampule is broken a few drops of the Kryptopyrrole should be distributed in several ampules sealed under nitrogen and stored in the freezer. For preparation of the standard an appropriate amount is weighed and dissolved in 1% aqueous ascorbic acid solution. This stock solution is stable for 72 hours if kept in the cold.

3. For preservation of the KP, ascorbic acid should be added to the freshly obtained urine (approximately several hundred mgm).
4. Porphobilinogen, which gives the same color reaction, will not interfere, as its complex with the Ehrlich's reagent is chloroform insoluble.

Obviously the presence of KP is not a diagnostic test for schizophrenia or for any known diagnostic group. But it does select a group of people who are all homogeneous with respect to the presence of the abnormal chemical in their urine. This "new" disease is caused by the excess formation in the body of products which are excreted as KP. These products, including KP, bind pyridoxine and zinc, producing a double dependency. Clinically they resemble the majority of schizophrenics no matter what criterion one uses to make the comparisons. I think we should use this diagnostic term "kryptopyrroluria" or simply pyrroluria as developed by Dr Pfeiffer, but it will take decades to break the tradition of using the old clinical diagnosis, useful many years ago, no longer useful, even detrimental to the health of the patients who are said to have it.

WORKS CITED

Altschul, R.; Hoffer, A., and Stephen, J.D. "Influence of nicotinic acid on serum cholesterol." *Archives of Biochemistry and Biophysics*, 54 (1955): 558-559.

American Psychiatric Association. *Task Force Report 7: Megavitamin and Orthomolecular Therapy in Psychiatry*. Washington, D.C., American Psychiatric Association, 1973

Conolly, J. *An Enquiry Concerning the Indications of Insanity 1830*. Rpt; London, England: Dawsons of Pall Mall, 1964.

Cott, A. *Fasting: The Ultimate Diet*. New York: Bantam Books, 1975.

Hoffer, A.; Osmond, H.; Callbeck, M.J.; and Kahan, I. "Treatment of schizophrenia with nicotinic acid and nicotinamide." *Journal of Clinical and Experimental Psychopathology*, 18 (1957): 131-158, 1957.

Hoffer, A. and Osmond, H. "Malvaria: a new psychiatric disease." *Acta Psychiatrica Scandanavia*, 39 (1963): 335-366.

Hoffer, A. and Osmond, H. *How To Live with Schizophrenia*. New York: University Books, Inc., 1966,, 1978.

Osmond, H. and Hoffer, A. "Schizophrenia and suicide." *Journal of Schizophrenia*, 1 (1967): 54-64.

Hoffer, A. "Five California schizophrenics." *Journal of Schizophrenia*, 1 (1967): 209-220.

Hoffer, A. and Osmond, H.: "In Reply to the American Psychiatric Association Task Force Report on Megavitamins and Orthomolecular Therapy in Psychiatry." Burnaby, BC: Canadian Schizophrenia Foundation, 1976.

Hoffer, A. *Common Questions About Schizophrenia and Their Answers*. New Canaan, CT: Keats Publishing, Inc., 1988.

Hoffer, A. *Orthomolecular Medicine for Physicians*. New Canaan, CT: Keats Publishing, Inc., 1989.

Hoffer, A. *Hoffer's Laws of Natural Nutrition: Eating Well for Pure Health.*. Kingston, ON: Quarry Press, 1996.

Hoffer, A. and Pauling, L. *Vitamin C and Cancer: Discovery, Recovery, and Controversy*. Kingston, ON: Quarry Press, 1998.

Hoffer, A. *Dr Hoffer's Guide to Natural Nutrition for Children*. Kingston, ON: Quarry Press, 1998.

Horrobin, D.F. *Omega 6 Essential Fatty Acids Pathophysiology and Role in Clinical Medicine.* New York: Alan R. Liss, 1990.

Huggins, H. "Mercury: a factor in mental disease." *Journal Orthomolecular Psychiatry,* 11 (1982): 3-16.

Jaffe, R. *Elisa/ACT™ Program Information Handbook.* Smithsburg, MD: Health Studies Collegium, 1987.

Kaufman, W. *Common Form of Niacinamide Deficiency Disease: Aniacinamidosis.* New Haven, CT: Yale University Press, 1943.

Kaufman, W. *The Common Form of Joint Dysfunction: Its Incidence and Treatment.* Brattleboro, VT: E. L. Hildreth and Co., 1949.

Kunin R.A. "Manganese and niacin in the treatment of drug-induced dyskinesias." *Journal of Orthomolecular Psychiatry,* 5 (1976): 4-27.

Lewis, N.D.C. and Pietrowski, Z.A. "Clinical diagnoses of manic-depressive psychosis." In *Depression.* Eds. Hoch, P.H. and Zubw, J. New York: Grune & Stratton, 1954.

Mandell, M. and Scanlon, L.W. *Dr Mandell's 5-Day Allergy Relief System.* New York: Thomas Y. Crowell, 1979.

Osmond, H. and Smythies, J. "Schizophrenia: a new approach." *Journal of Mental Science,* 98 (1952): 309-315.

Pauling, L.: "Orthomolecular psychiatry." *Science,* 160 (1968): 265-271.

Pauling, L. *Vitamin C and the Common Cold.* NY: W.H. Freeman & Co., 197?.

Pauling, L. *How To Live Longer and Feel Better.* New York, NY: W.H. Freeman & Co., 1986.

Pfeiffer, C.C.; Sohler, A.; Jenney, M.S., and Iliev, V. "Treatment of pyrroluric schizophrenia (malvaria) with large doses of pyridoxine and a dietary supplement of zinc." *Journal of Applied Nutrition,* 26 (1974): 21-28.

Philpott, W.H. "Maladaptive reactions to frequently used foods and commonly met chemicals as precipitating factors in many chronic physical and chronic emotional illnesses." In *A Physicians Handbook on Orthomolecular Medicine.* Eds. R. J. Williams and D.K. Kalita. New Canaan, CT: Keats Publishing, Inc. 1979.

Rudin, D.O. "The dominant diseases of modernized societies as Omega-3 essential fatty acid deficiency syndrome: substrate beri beri." *Medical Hypothesis,* 8 (1982): 17-47.

Slagle P: *The Way Up From Down.* New York, NY: Random House, 1987.

Stone, I. *The Healing Factor: Vitamin C Against Disease.* New York, NY: Grosset and Dunlap, 1972.

Wittenborn, J.R.: "A search for responders to niacin supplementation." *Archives of General Psychiatry,* 31 (1974): 547-552.

ACKNOWLEDGEMENTS

I thank Bob Hilderley and his staff at Quarry Press for publishing this book when no one else would, and secondly for his remarkable editing and restructuring of the original manuscript.

When in 1967 I left my two jobs in Saskatchewan, Associate Professor of Psychiatry and Director of Psychiatric Research, Department of Health, Psychiatric Services Branch, Saskatchewan, I took with me a mass of clinical data dealing with our clinical studies of the treatment of schizophrenia using the orthomolecular program. This data summarized the results of our early pioneer studies, our clinical studies and the double blind controlled studies — the first in world psychiatry. The clinical files on which this data was based are housed in the Hoffer Archives (Saskatchewan Archives Board, Murray Building, University of Saskatchewan, 3 Campus Drive, Saskatoon SK S7N 5A4)

The patient files of these prospective randomized double blind controlled trials are stored in this archive. Much of this material has been summarized and reported, but most was not because it was too voluminous and because it was impossible to get medical and psychiatric journals interested. After the first few papers had been published and after the controversy became strident and vigorous, we were shut out of the psychiatric and medical journals.

About six years ago I began to sort this data and to prepare a comprehensive report. At the same time I had collaborated with Linus Pauling in several reports on the treatment of cancer using nutrients, primarily vitamin C in large doses. After I had treated about 45 patients it was clear that the patients receiving this program were living longer than the ones who would not or could not do so. This was the beginning of corroboration of the work of Ewan Cameron and Linus Pauling published years earlier.

At a Festchrift for Arthur Sackler attended by Linus Pauling, I stayed in a small motel next door to Linus. The first morning I visited him and told him about these preliminary results. He was impressed and intrigued, and asked whether I planned to publish. I replied that I did not. When he asked why not, I replied that I was certain I could not find anyone who would. He then asked me to collect what data I had, let him see it, and he would find a publisher for it. I did not take this too seriously, thinking he was being generous to me and encouraging.

However, two years later when I had not done anything except add many more patients to the series, I received a letter from Dr Pauling asking me where the data was. This spurred me into action and I reviewed the outcome of the treatment of 134 patients with cancer, seen over a ten year period between 1978 and 1988. We published this material. Later we agreed to publish a book by Hoffer and Pauling. I had suggested it should be Pauling and Hoffer but he would not hear of that. He completed his portion and I had completed most of mine, but eventually he could not find anyone to publish. This was very unusual because until then he had not had difficulty finding publishers for his marvellous books. But even The New York Academy of Sciences would not accept his clinical views, even though by tradition they never rejected papers written by their members. There was no Honorary MD among his 45 PhDs and DScs.

Facing this stalemate I talked to my son Bill about our publishing dilemma. He suggested that I contact Bob Hilderley. He said that he had dealt with Bob in connection with his Tanks series of books and had found him friendly, a good editor, and honest. Quarry Press was small, but I thought that a small publisher who would publish was preferable to spending years trying to find a major one, most of whom would not.

Bob expressed interest and I submitted this manuscript and several others to him. He was willing to take it on when no other publisher would because the use of vitamins in treating cancer was too far out. It was a new and strange and perhaps fearful paradigm that no publisher wanted to enter. At the same time I submitted the schizophrenia/vitamin B-3 manuscript and later a manuscript on the treatment of children. By then, he had already published my first Quarry book, *Hoffers Laws*. I liked what he had done and now trusted him fully.

He re-wrote and restructured this book with great art and understanding of science. The work is seamless, and unless I compare this manuscript with the one I sent him, I am not sure which was mine unchanged, which is his unchanged, and which is a skillful editing of mine and his.

To my surprise I found the book interesting again. Usually after I complete a work I find it difficult and disinteresting to read it again. But this time I was fascinated by what I had written, and what had been rewritten by Bob. I think it is a very good book and the data is correct. If only physicians will read and think about it.

The mass of clinical data I have accumulated since 1967 in Saskatoon and since 1976 in Victoria fully supports the conclusions in this book.

May 19, 1998　　　　　　　　　　A. Hoffer MD PhD FRCP(C)

QUARRY HEALTH BOOKS

How To Live with Schizophrenia
Abram Hoffer with Dr Humphry Osmond
$19.95 CDA/$14.95 USA

*Common Questions about Schizophrenia
and Their Answers*
Dr Abram Hoffer $19.95 CDA/$14.95 USA

*Hoffer's Laws of Natural Nutrition:
A Guide to Eating Well for Pure Health*
Dr Abram Hoffer $19.95 CDA /$14.95 USA

*Dr Hoffer's A,B,C of
Natural Nutrition for Children*
Dr Abram Hoffer $19.95 CDA / $14.95 USA

*Vitamin C & Cancer:
Discovery, Recover, Controversy*
Dr Abram Hoffer with Linus Pauling
$16.95 CDA / $12.95 USA

*The Botanical Pharmacy:
A Resource for Health-Care Professionals*
by Heather Boon and Michael Smith
$39.95 CDA / $29.95 USA

*Women's Naturopathic Medicine:
Maternal Naturopathic Care*
by Lisa Doran $34.95 CDA / $26.95 USA

*Lifting the Bull:
Back Pain, Fibromyalgia, and Environmental Illness*
by Diane Dawber $18.95 CDA / $14.95 USA

*Reading To Heal:
A Reading Group Strategy for Better Health*
by Diane Dawber $9.95 CDA / $6.95 USA

Available at your favorite bookstore or directly from Quarry Health Books,
P.O. Box 1061, Kingston, Ontario, Canada K7L 4Y5, Tel (613) 548-8429,
Fax. (613) 548-1556, E-mail: order@quarrypress.com